The Essential Guide to

Alzheimer's

ROBERT DUFFY SERIES EDITOR

Published in Great Britain in 2019 by
need2know
Remus House
Coltsfoot Drive
Peterborough
PE2 9BF
Telephone 01733 898103
www.need2knowbooks.co.uk

Contents

Introduction

While attitudes are changing towards Alzheimer's, the initial vision which springs to mind is likely to be a pretty negative one. As of 2019, there were 850,000 people in the UK living with dementia, a number set to increase to over a million by 2025. The most common type of dementia is Alzheimer's disease, which affects 62% of dementia sufferers – that's around 527,000 people. Being diagnosed with Alzheimer's is life changing.

But these 527,000 people aren't the only ones affected by Alzheimer's. It affects people who treat the person – whether for Alzheimer's or for indirect medical conditions. Friends, children, partners or spouses of people suffering from Alzheimer's are all affected too. Those in regular contact with the person, and those who care for them every day, all need to live with the effects of this condition. Many will want to learn all they can on the subject and some will want it in simple, easy to understand terms.

Anyone who has an interest in the disease and anyone who is affected by it either directly or indirectly can benefit from this book. Our main goal here is to answer any questions a newly diagnosed, or even an undiagnosed person might have while maintaining a focus on the experience of the Alzheimer's patient. We now know more than ever before about the disease and how it affects the brain. New drugs are coming out all the time and research is constantly underway to both find a cure and to better understand the disease.

The average progression of the condition takes between eight and 12 years, and at present there's no cure. That said, the outlook for people with this condition is becoming increasingly more positive as time goes on, with developments being made in the area all the time. Our understanding of the condition and the care being offered to those living with it are slowly developing as our attitudes change. People living with Alzheimer's disease are getting to live better, fuller lives as we learn more about how to prepare for the progression of the disease, and how caregivers should be trained in order to provide the best medical attention possible.

When the late Terry Pratchett stood up and publicly announced that he was in the early stages of Alzheimer's, he did the Alzheimer's community a massive favour. In doing this, he helped us understand that Alzheimer's is a disease that large numbers of people are currently living with (not dying from!), and that the condition is not something to be ashamed of.

We're writing this book under the assumption that anyone who reads it will know someone who is – or will themselves be – in the early stages of the disease, either suspecting that they are about to be diagnosed or trying to get information about their condition following diagnosis. This is because this, unsurprisingly, is when most people begin to educate themselves about Alzheimer's disease.

All the same, even if you're in a later stage of the condition, this book will come in handy in educating you about the progression you can expect the disease to make and allowing you to plan for the future.

You're likely to have a lot of questions right now: What do I do now? Why do I have this disease? What should I have done to avoid this? What do I say to my friends and family?

On a different level, other queries may come up: What medication is available and what will it do? What's the difference between dementia and Alzheimer's? What does this condition actually do to a brain?

This book sets out to help you deal with these questions, which are likely to be your first thoughts on receiving your diagnosis.

Many of the questions addressed will also be ones which family and friends will have and this book is also written with these in mind. A specific focus on these questions can be found in Chapters 9 and 10.

This book will also come in handy to professionals working with people with Alzheimer's disease. Whether you're a member of staff in a care home, an occupational therapist, a nurse or anyone else who works with Alzheimer's patients, there'll be something in it for you.

Although the actions of a person with Alzheimer's can appear random, there are often fascinating reasons behind them. For instance, it might seem as though someone has picked up a sudden hatred for cauliflower and potatoes, but there are actually reasons for this which have been uncovered by scientific research. We have come a long way in the last 30 years and, with the research and development going on in the area, it cannot be ruled out that a cure may be found in our lifetime.

The professional care of a person with Alzheimer's can be improved if we understand why these changes take place. This book will go a long way towards you gaining that knowledge, whether you or your partner suffer from the condition. Approaching Alzheimer's disease positively and without fear is by far the best way of coping with the condition.

A positive attitude can only really come from knowledge of what it is the future holds.

Disclaimer

If you suspect that you have Alzheimer's, it is important to consult a healthcare professional and obtain a proper diagnosis. This book is not intended to replace professional medical advice – it was written to provide general information on Alzheimer's disease only. Following an Alzheimer's diagnosis, it's important that you follow any advice given to you by your GP and other healthcare professionals over any other sources.

National guidelines and recommendations can change, so it is important to check with your GP or healthcare professional before acting on any of the information in this book. At the time of going to press, all the information featured in this book was correct.

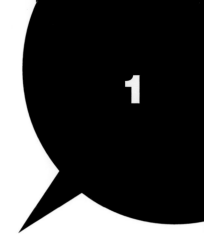

1

Alzheimer's in the Past

I t does seem to be a transient time for Alzheimer's and this becomes more apparent when you look back 20 or 30 years to what life used to be like for sufferers. From steps being taken towards a cure to scientists discovering more about what causes Alzheimer's and figuring out new ways to treat or prevent it, Alzheimer's seems to constantly be in the news today.

Not so long ago, knowledge of how to help and make life easier for someone with Alzheimer's was practically non-existent, and it was easiest to just take the stance that "Granny's gone a bit mad" and "there's nothing we can do". We've really come a long way over the last few years.

What We Used to Believe

Right into the 1950s, the general understanding was that any mental illness an old person might experience was a result of anxiety, schizophrenia, depression, senility or something more extreme, and that dementia would always be the result.

A neurologist was generally required to make a diagnosis of Alzheimer's, and this was done by ruling out other causes of dementia like brain tumours, vitamin B12 deficiencies, alcoholism and syphilis.

A hopeless picture was still presented of the conditions commonly referred to as "degenerative dementia" in the 1980s. Little or no thought was put into keeping the mind active or into slowing the progress of the disease. Treatment mostly involved allowing the disease to take its course while dealing with only the individual's most basic needs. "Senile dementia" was a term often used 20 years ago and it was seen just as an accepted part of growing old.

Over the last 50 years, the very words we use to describe dementia have changed entirely.

Over the last 50 years, the very words we use to describe dementia have changed entirely.

What Did a Diagnosis Mean?

Care for those with Alzheimer's or dementia was left to family members in the 1950s, as no treatment was available. When it did occur, it tended to be hushed up and dealt with in the best way the family could. There was still a lot of guesswork going on and a lot of ignorance surrounding the disease. If someone's behaviour was considered very disturbed – if they were unable to cook, clean and look after themselves – and they had no family available to support them, mental hospital was the only option.

Admittance to these hospitals, even in these extreme cases, really depended on whether or not someone was able to convince local psychiatrists that it was necessary. A paper detailing the outcomes after elderly people were admitted to stay at a mental hospital for two years was published in 1955 by Martin Roth. Those categorised as "dements" had mainly died, while those with acute confusional states had either recovered or died, with a 50/50 split on this.

It was found that those who were diagnosed as schizophrenics were kept in the hospital, while those with symptoms of depression on admission were mostly already discharged after two years. From this study, Roth concluded that only those with dementia symptoms had significant brain disease, while other various symptoms could have more than one cause.

Alzheimer's was not a subject which was discussed by the vast majority of the population, as a fear of the unknown existed.

When Did Things Get Better?

Over time, psychogeriatric units began to open, with Roth's research gradually leading to a more positive attitude towards Alzheimer's disease. Roth opened a research unit in 1962 to examine the relationship between mental breakdown and physical disease.

In addition, Roth recruited Dr Gary Blessed to examine the patients while hospitalised, establish a diagnosis and assess their cognitive functioning capabilities.

Responsible for 87% of the cases he studied, Blessed discovered that the most common pathology was Alzheimer's disease. This finding briefly led to the belief that all cases of dementia in old age had to be Alzheimer's. However, this was later proven untrue through further research.

The idea that psychotherapy could help people with dementia was quite foreign, even as late as the 1980s. The general assumption was that the retentive powers of memory necessary for therapy to be successful were entirely absent in those with Alzheimer's. It has been discovered, however, that people with dementia are far more resourceful than once thought, so several forms of therapeutic work are now being explored.

What's Different Today?

In the 1970s and 1980s, special psychogeriatric units began to spring up all over the UK, but they were not universal. In many respects, the 1980s are seen as a key decade in the history of Alzheimer's. With a growing awareness of the disease, gradual change has been possible. This change allowed the number of psychogeriatricians – specialists in the field of mental health in later life – to increase, and made it possible for diagnosis, treatment and management services for the elderly mentally ill to improve thanks to lobbying within the Royal College of Psychiatrists.

In 1988 a public talk was given to raise the profile of old age psychiatry, but ignorance still remained about the disease. Alzheimer's continued to be described as "the silent epidemic" throughout the decade.

Eventually, organisations like the Alzheimer's Society were founded and people had somewhere they could turn to for advice and support. Alzheimer's was slowly becoming a subject that could be talked about openly.

The increase in people living longer has resulted in Alzheimer's becoming an issue which cannot be ignored. A number of aspects of Alzheimer's care, such as diagnoses and drugs, are being improved greatly every day, and this all comes down to the original research some 40 years ago. The changes in demographics have certainly made this an increasingly urgent topic, although medicine and science were gradually converging to see it as one.

What Can We Expect Today?

The specialist psychogeriatric units which began to spring up in the 1970s and 1980s have now been replaced by specialist nursing homes. While the money invested is still not enough, it does signify a big change in attitudes, and progress is being made. Alzheimer's is now being discussed instead of hushed up, and people are being diagnosed much earlier, allowing more time to respond to drugs and treatment.

Over the last 30 to 40 years, and especially since the 1980s, a great deal has changed. Attitudes from medical professionals, in particular GPs, are slowly but surely changing as knowledge is greater. The stigma surrounding Alzheimer's disease is slowly disappearing as the condition becomes more common and more is understood about it. Patients with Alzheimer's now have so many more options than just mental hospital or family care.

GPs are now able to diagnose at an earlier stage when help can be given and plans can be made. Efforts are still being made to learn more about how to prevent and treat Alzheimer's, as it's no longer viewed as an inevitable part of growing old.

One common problem in the later stages of Alzheimer's is falling, which is the most frequent and serious type of accident to occur in those aged 65 and over. In order to raise national recognition of this problem, Help the Aged have started a National Falls Awareness Day.

As recently as 25 years ago, GPs were only diagnosing Alzheimer's when symptoms had become undeniably obvious and the patients themselves were no longer manageable for their family and friends. Some were misdiagnosed altogether.

The government announced in December 2008 that training on how to recognise the early symptoms of Alzheimer's would be given to all NHS GPs in England. This followed a survey which found that only 31% of GPs felt they had received adequate training to manage and diagnose the condition. Such action should lead to GPs being better placed to refer patients on to organisations which can help and provide support.

More recently, the Alzheimer's Society launched a free online programme in partnership with BMJ learning, targeted at GPs, GP trainees and practice nurses. This course has sections dealing with non-drug treatments to address behavioural problems, early diagnosis and basic information about dementia.

Even though there is plenty of help out there, Alzheimer's organisations rarely receive requests from GPs for more information on what support they can provide, and patients rarely receive this information from their GPs.

Case Studies

Alzheimer's in the 1980s

In 1981, Alan's mother was diagnosed with Alzheimer's at the age of 66.

"We started noticing changes in my mum around two years before she was diagnosed. We were becoming increasingly concerned about her – she ran a small business and was starting to have problems handling money. She was doing things that were really out of character, and her sense of judgement and reasoning was becoming strained.

"My mum had been hit by the bombings in the war, so after a number of visits to the GP he concluded that it was just an old war wound. He said it was an unavoidable part of growing old.

"When she finally received the correct diagnosis, nobody told me and my mum kept it a secret. At one point, I visited the GP and the receptionist said, "I was so sorry to hear about your mum." When she realised I didn't know what she was talking about, she started to backtrack and wouldn't tell me what was wrong with my mum.

"Eventually, things got so bad that the GP had no choice but to tell me about my mother's dementia. Even then, he kept using phrases like "all part of old age" and "just a little confused". The doctor accused me of doing my mother's hair and making sure she was well presented to "cover up" how sick she was. He insisted it would be best if I just left her alone so they could section her under the Mental Health Act, because my assistance had stopped them from doing a proper assessment of her earlier."

Even though there is plenty of help out there, Alzheimer's organisations rarely receive requests from GPs for more information on what support they can provide, and patients rarely receive this information from their GPs.

The problems didn't end when hospital care came. Several health problems were misdiagnosed, with Alan being told he was overreacting, and staff appeared ignorant of his mother's needs and lacked sensitivity. The hospital decided to transfer Alan's mother to somewhere more secure after she wandered out of the psychiatric hospital in her slippers.

It was a long, hard struggle for Alan's family, but care did eventually improve and his mother did settle down.

Today's Treatment

Beth was diagnosed with Alzheimer's three years ago, when she was 72.

"I started having difficulty with word-finding around the year 2000. I was used to doing a lot of public speaking and was increasingly forgetting words and phrases. I was working as a university lecturer at this stage. My symptoms had just started becoming more apparent when I was elected as a local authority councillor.

"I got so used to people not believing me about the problems that I delayed visiting the doctor until three years ago. A diagnosis of Alzheimer's was made following referrals to a psychiatrist, a psychologist and a neurologist, and three different types of brain scan.

"I hadn't expected it even though I had felt it in my bones. The diagnosis surprised me. I have tried two different types of medication since then, but neither agreed with me unfortunately.

"I was told that there was nothing else to be done for me pretty soon after my diagnosis. I felt dumped by the system – the disappointment hit me pretty hard. But a massive change came when a neighbour told me about Alzheimer's Scotland. That group was able to put me in contact with the Scottish Dementia Working Group. They have given me all sorts of books and information. The two organisations have been amazingly helpful. They visit me at home and I know I can call them if I need to. They've shown me where I can go if I need help, and explained lots of things about my condition which I didn't understand before.

"Most importantly, I continue to enjoy my life socialising with friends. Things have become easier now that I've learned how to adapt my life to my condition. I'm getting so much more comfortable with asking for help."

Summing Up

- We have come a long way from the attitudes of the 1950s when Alzheimer's was seen as inevitable, though we still have a long way to go when it comes to the treatment of people with Alzheimer's. We're still working to improve diagnosis, care and long term treatment.

- Apart from dealing with their basic needs, the view of people with Alzheimer's as recently as 1980 was that there was nothing that we could do.

- Dr Gary Blessed and Dr Martin Roth conducted significant research in this area, with their research findings leading to more being known about Alzheimer's and a change in attitudes.

- Many see the 1980s as a key decade for Alzheimer's research. This is when elderly mental health became a branch of the Royal College of Psychiatrists in its own right for the first time.

- Although we've achieved a lot in the last few years, a lot of people feel that after their diagnosis, they're somewhat abandoned by the healthcare system. Hopefully, we can work to end that by ensuring that all GPs are given more training on the subject.

- As mental hospitals have shut, more specialist care homes have sprung up and the stigma surrounding Alzheimer's is no longer so prevalent.

- This is seen in the changes in terminology used. It is now rare to hear the phrases "degenerative dementia" or "senile dementia".

2

What is Alzheimer's Disease?

Many people believe that dementia and Alzheimer's are the same thing because the terms are used interchangeably so often. They may even appear the same to an outsider looking at the symptoms and development. All the same, it's a good idea to have an understanding of how the two are connected and what the differences are.

The Medical Definition

Dementia is an umbrella term to describe a serious deterioration in mental function such as memory, language, orientation and judgement. Alzheimer's disease is one type of dementia. Affecting over 500,000 people in the UK, it accounts for 62% of dementia cases, making it the most common type. So it is quite understandable that people will get the terms dementia and Alzheimer's mixed up.

The symptoms are similar and much of the advice given with regards to Alzheimer's is valid for other forms of dementia. The second most common is vascular dementia (also known as multi-infarct dementia), followed by dementia with Lewy bodies and fronto-temporal dementia. Dementia comes in an estimated 50 to 100 different types. As the effects of a culture rife with binge-drinking take their toll, one form of dementia – Korsakoff's syndrome, or alcohol related dementia – is also becoming increasingly common.

Most people will have no need to distinguish what type it is when they meet someone who has dementia.

All the same, it's useful to have an understanding of why certain changes occur, how Alzheimer's differs from other forms of dementia and how it affects the brain if we want to understand what Alzheimer's is and how it affects us.

Let's Go Back In Time

We'll begin with a short history lesson on how Alzheimer's was first discovered in order to understand more about this condition.

Dr Alois Alzheimer was a German psychiatrist and neuropathologist, and the condition Alzheimer's is named after him. He became fascinated by a patient in her fifties who showed a number of behavioural symptoms including short term memory loss during his work at the start of the 20th century. He had her medical notes and brain sent to his lab when she died in 1906.

Dr Alzheimer, alongside his two Italian colleagues, examined the brain and found that it had decreased in size. The death of a large number of nerve cells appeared to be the cause. They used a microscope to look inside the dying cells, and saw unusual plaques which were made up partly of brain cells and tangles. Alzheimer presented a key paper at the South West German Society of Alienists on the 3rd of November 1906. It took less than five years for these research findings to be used to diagnose patients in Germany and abroad.

Alzheimer's disease was largely ignored for the first few decades of the 20th century. The research started moving once again, however, when scientists in the 1970s discovered that some parts of the brain were shrinking more than others, and that particular types of nerve cells were becoming more damaged – these were the temporal lobes at the side of the brain, which are responsible for storing recent memories.

So What's the Difference?

To understand better, here are some brief details on the main types of dementia other than Alzheimer's. It is worth noting that there are some differences in symptoms between Alzheimer's and other types of dementia, though many of the symptoms you experience will be similar to those of most other types.

- **Vascular dementia** occurs when oxygen supply to the brain is affected by damage to blood cells. This can result in brain cells dying, which in turn can lead to a series of mini strokes. Each stroke will destroy a small number of brain cells by cutting off its blood supply, even though externally the strokes are so light that you might not even notice them. Vascular dementia occurs as a result of this damage.

  - If you have vascular dementia, your mental decline is likely to have a specific start date – usually a stroke (also known as a CVA or cerebral vascular accident). Because some areas of the brain may be more affected than others, sufferers may have some symptoms but not others. Rather than a gradual decline, symptoms will generally get worse in a series of steps.

  - Epilepsy, depression and mood swings are all common symptoms of vascular dementia. In some cases, Alzheimer's and vascular dementia can occur together.

- **Dementia with Lewy bodies** is named for an abnormal collection of proteins that can occur in the nerve cells of the brain, called Lewy bodies. This condition can affect the ability to reason and judge distances, as well as the concentration, memory, language and attention. More than half of those with Lewy bodies develop symptoms of Parkinson's disease, and some will also experience visual hallucinations.

- **Fronto-temporal dementia** often occurs to people in their forties or fifties – an earlier age than Alzheimer's disease. Like Alzheimer's disease, it involves a progressive decline in a person's mental abilities over the years, but damage to the brain cells is more localised than in Alzheimer's and the sufferer does not usually have lapses in memory. It gets its name from the frontal lobe of the brain, which is the area affected by the condition.

  - People with fronto-temporal dementia can often appear selfish and uncaring because the frontal lobe of the brain controls mood and behaviour, so those with the condition can become very fixed in their moods.

There are differences in symptoms between Alzheimer's and other types of dementia, though many of the symptoms you experience will be similar to those of most other types.

- **Korsakoff's syndrome** is dementia that's related to alcohol. The main symptom is short term memory loss but the person may also have difficulties in learning new skills. Often as a result of a poor diet, those with Korsakoff's are generally deficient in vitamin B1 (thiamine).

How Does Alzheimer's Affect the Brain?

The tangles and plaques which develop in the brain to cause Alzheimer's lead to a shortage of brain chemicals which are involved in transmitting messages within the brain, and to the death of brain cells. The condition is then made worse when the plaques and tangles start attacking other connections between brain cells.

Why Certain Changes Occur

Memory loss – usually short term memory loss – is one of the most commonly discussed symptoms of Alzheimer's disease. We don't actually know for sure why short term memories are affected more than long term memories, but one thought is that long term memories are more stable because they are stored in a different part of the brain and relearned many times.

The brain begins to shrink as more nerve cells die. As the brain starts to shrink and it has to rely on fewer chemical messengers, key mental skills start to diminish. This decreased size is what first caught Dr Alzheimer's eye back in the early 20th century.

Changes to Expect

Symptoms may include mood swings, forgetting recent events, names and faces, becoming confused when handling money or driving a car and problems with language. Memory loss is likely to become worse as the disease progresses, moving from occasional difficulties accessing short-term memories to more frequent memory loss, and eventually loss of longer-term memories too.

In the advanced stages of the disease, loss of inhibitions and wandering off are also common symptoms.

Summing Up

- Dementia comes in a number of types, but Alzheimer's is the most common. The next four most-common types include Lewy bodies, Korsakoff's, fronto-temporal and vascular dementia.

- Plaques and tangles in the brain kill off brain cells and reduce the size of the brain, resulting in the symptoms of Alzheimer's.

- As the disease progresses, key brain functions will deteriorate.

- The disease was discovered by German psychiatrist and neuropathologist Dr Alois Alzheimer.

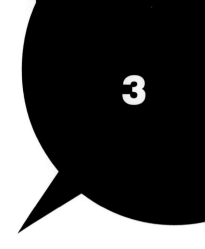

3

Signs of Alzheimer's Disease

A poll conducted by researchers Millward Brown in 2004 found that out of six European countries, the UK had, on average, the longest time between first symptoms being noticed and a diagnosis of Alzheimer's being made (32 months). This is almost twice the amount of time a diagnosis takes in France, Spain, Poland, Italy and Germany where it takes just 18 months to be diagnosed. Many years may pass between the time you, your family or friends notice that something is wrong, and the time you get a diagnosis. It can be a real journey.

Why Does Diagnosis Take So Long?

Experts do agree that treatment for Alzheimer's is more effective if it begins in the early stages. So why is there such a delay here in Britain? Why are we stuck at 32 months when other countries can do it in 18? The researchers who ran the poll suggested that it's not so much an issue with our medical system as with our national attitude – rather than looking for help, we delay and hope the symptoms will go away.

We refuse to make a fuss and choose, instead, to ignore the problem. It is a hard disease to diagnose and we tend to assume that we will become more forgetful as we get older. Another theory suggests that the symptoms of Alzheimer's are simply assumed to be pointing at a different condition. The difficulty lies in working out which forgetfulness is just a natural part of aging and which is an indicator that the individual is developing dementia.

How do you know that it is Alzheimer's? Next, we're going to take a look at the early symptoms you should be watching out for.

The difficulty lies in working out which forgetfulness is just a natural part of aging and which is an indicator that the individual is developing dementia.

Alzheimer's Early Warning Signs

While symptoms can vary between individuals, a diagnosis of Alzheimer's will involve looking for the most common early symptoms. Symptoms may initially be so subtle that they are not noted. The fact that the symptoms of Alzheimer's can often be mistaken for something else is a big part of the reason diagnosis takes so long, as we've already discussed.

Other conditions like urinary tract infections (UTI) and depression should always be ruled out first. A confused state can sometimes happen as a result of both of these conditions, and both can cause forgetfulness. The doctor should also take note of whether the symptoms have been getting worse, and how long they've been going on for.

Forgetting Things

In the early stages, it is short term memory as opposed to long term memory which is affected – forgetting what you did yesterday or going upstairs for something and then forgetting why you were going up. This symptom fits in with the stereotypical image people have of sufferers, and is probably the most well known of the early symptoms of Alzheimer's.

It tends to take longer for childhood memories and long-term events to be affected, as they appear to be stored in a different part of the brain.

Getting Words Confused

We can all forget what we were about to say halfway through a sentence, but sometimes this can be a sign of a greater underlying issue. This may just seem like regular forgetfulness at times, but as cognitive functions begin to become impaired it may begin to demonstrate a more troubling lack of coherency.

Mixing Up Places, People and Times

In the early stages, this may be as simple as going to an appointment on the wrong day or perhaps turning up more than once. As the disease progresses, this can evolve into mixing up family members (e.g. recognising a mother's face but thinking she's her daughter), or going back to a childhood home thinking you still live there. In many cases, this is the symptom which triggers people to finally take action.

Struggling to Carry Out Familiar Tasks

Tasks which have been performed for years such as putting on the washing machine may slide from the memory. Tasks around the house can start becoming difficult. Handling money can also become a challenge, and you may forget how to figure out how much money to hand over when shopping.

Personality Changes

You may become anxious, changing from being a calm and collected person to becoming an anxious one. In many cases, you and the people around you won't quite be able to pin down what exactly has changed. Inhibitions may come out in strange or inappropriate ways, and feelings of paranoia may appear.

Altered Behaviour and Mood

Many doctors will misdiagnose this symptom. For example, you might be diagnosed with depression if your mood becomes depressed, even though your mood is just another symptom of this bigger condition.

Losing Things

Some people will start hiding things all over the house for no apparent reason, or start putting things in the fridge even though they don't belong there.

Lack of Motivation

This is a common symptom of depression, but can also be a sign of Alzheimer's. It's worth investigating if someone who was once very active gives up their favourite hobbies and starts spending hours in front of the TV.

How Does Alzheimer's Develop?

This question is a little more difficult to answer. There are no guides on how the disease will develop beyond the first few symptoms. This can be frustrating as comfort can be gained from knowing what to expect. Nobody can give a timescale or foresee what the future holds, though we can say that Alzheimer's generally involves a more gradual decline than other forms of dementia, with changes happening over time rather in steep steps.

What we can say is that every individual case progresses at a different rate. While some people may go downhill rapidly, others will stay at the same level for a long time. We also know that doctors are able to do more to slow down the disease's progression if it is diagnosed early on. There's more time to organise activities that can keep the brain active, and to try different medications to find one that works.

Other Signs that It Is Progressing

Some signs exist that will tell you whether or not the Alzheimer's is progressing. Friends and family sometimes first notice that symptoms have worsened when the person begins to revert back to the past, thinking today is yesteryear. Maybe you'll find that you're unable to do things that you could do just a few months ago. Two further symptoms include losing weight unexpectedly, or forgetting to take your medication. If someone is eating enough but continuing to lose weight, this can be a symptom of Alzheimer's. Alternatively, it could be an indicator that the individual has forgotten how to cook or isn't eating properly.

When Should We Call the Doctor?

If you have a hunch that something just isn't right, or if family and friends have started to notice and point things out, it is time to seek advice. You need to talk to someone as early as possible if you think you or someone you love has Alzheimer's.

Many people are surprised at how little is done by the GP. When it comes to accessing services, your GP is the best person to speak to as they can act as a point of contact between you and the specialists. If there are problems with behaviour, like aggression, a referral can be made to a psychiatrist. Your doctor will want to rule out any conditions where your body is full of toxins – like a UTI (urinary tract infection) or chest infection – and any other mental illnesses – like depression – before suggesting that dementia could be the cause. Beyond that, there's little they can do to treat the condition as a whole – they'll have to focus on working with the smaller issues that Alzheimer's can cause. However, if the Alzheimer's is not causing any problems, the GP is unlikely to suggest action. Brain scans are not routinely performed and a diagnosis will usually be given based on behaviour and changes over time.

A referral from your GP can allow social workers to get involved if you need any help with your daily needs.

It's not likely that an Alzheimer's diagnosis will be made with certainty, even after the leaps in treatment and diagnosis we've experienced in recent years.

Questions to Ask

For the majority of questions that spring to mind immediately following diagnosis, there will be no answer: How long do I have? How long will I go on like this? Why did I have to get this disease? How quickly will the changes happen? Although it's understandable to want to know these answers, your GP won't be able to help you here.

More practical questions will crop up when you've had more time to think: How can I keep as well as possible? What should I be doing? It is also worth asking about local services and what is available to help you keep your brain active, such as mind clinics, support groups and daycare. The information is there and help is available. Most drugs are most effective earlier on, so it's also best to ask about medication as soon as possible.

We should note here that your GP won't always be the best source of information at this point. Things are slowly improving, but for now it's best to ask as many of your questions as possible to specialists in psychiatry or social work, or an organisation that specialises in Alzheimer's.

I've Been Diagnosed: What Now?

If it is considered that further health or social work services are required, a needs assessment may be carried out in the home by either a social worker or a community psychiatric nurse (CPN). The idea is that it should flag up any problem areas. The questions asked will be thorough and will go through all aspects of your daily living skills: how you get about, whether you socialise much, if you wear glasses, if you need to see a chiropodist, if you have any problems with incontinence, if you are able to wash yourself and if you have any other physical ailments.

What happens after diagnosis will depend on whether your healthcare providers think you'd currently benefit from further support. In order to make a decision, a needs assessment is necessary to gather as much information as possible.

These assessments often go on for a while as they need to cover every aspect of your life – what services you need, whether your home will need any adaptations or aids, and what you get up to during the day.

Other Areas of Help

Without a doubt, you'll be looking for sources of support following your diagnosis. There are loads of different organisations worth considering.

Support Groups

Here you can meet with others in the same situation, talk about your worries, share experiences and discuss how to deal with things. Support groups are often run by groups like the Alzheimer's Society or Alzheimer's Scotland. They're pretty informal and usually run around once a month. Many people find it really helpful to know that there are other people out there in the same situation as them, and support groups can also be a great place to share information about local services and what there is available near you.

Alzheimer's Scotland and The Alzheimer's Society

They can provide information and leaflets on various aspects of the disease and give advice on what help there is available, as well as providing valuable services like support groups, drop in cafes and befrienders. Alzheimer's Scotland and the Alzheimer's Society can provide advice, support and assistance that isn't always available elsewhere, and many people with Alzheimer's have described them as lifesavers for this reason.

For contact details, check the help list at the back of this book.

Daycare Centres

Accessing a daycare centre generally requires a referral from your GP or social worker. These organisations will generally be run by your local health board. A daycare centre will encourage activities that keep your mind active and allow any further assessment deemed necessary. Beginning with a morning snack and drink, the day is then filled with various group activities: discussing current news events, card making, general knowledge quizzes, ball games for coordination, basic colouring in, baking groups, reminiscence boxes and group discussions where everyone is given the opportunity to talk about their favourite holidays, where they went to school or anything else about the past.

The setup will vary from centre to centre, but the aims remain the same. Those attending the daycare centre will get to choose what they want to get involved in, and there are usually loads of different activities to choose from.

A daycare centre will encourage activities that keep your mind active and allow any further assessment deemed necessary.

Home Visits

Social workers may visit regularly (if they feel you need it) and care workers may be assigned to help you with daily needs. Depending on your specific needs, home visits may be helpful to you. If you need help with behaviour, depression or anxiety, a CPN may visit you for a short period.

Summing Up

- Treatment is generally more effective the earlier a diagnosis is made.

- Before getting a diagnosis of Alzheimer's, you first need to rule out other potential causes of your symptoms, so your GP should be your first port of call.

- While it may not be offered straight away, there is plenty of help and assistance available.

- The Alzheimer's Society and Alzheimer's Scotland are great for everything from information to regular support.

- Services are only usually offered if it is felt that there is a problem which needs to be treated.

- While symptoms do vary, there are several common first symptoms.

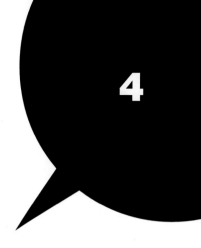

4

Can I Stop My Condition from Getting Worse?

Millions of pounds are spent each year researching Alzheimer's and its causes and possible cures. A "cure" or something to stop the disease's progression is often one of the first things a patient will ask about following diagnosis. You want to prevent the disease from worsening, and it's only natural that you'll ask for a cure that can do this.

Unfortunately, it seems as though it will take much more research and much more investment before we can hope to come up with a real cure. It's possible that we're just one step away from discovering a cure, and progress is being made, but we aren't there just yet.

We need to look at other issues – such as lifestyle – and work on these whether a cure is found in the near future or not. Having an active social life and keeping mentally and physically fit keeps the brain cells alive and can go a long way in slowing down the hold Alzheimer's has on the brain. There are very strong links between the progression of Alzheimer's and a patient's lifestyle.

Some early-stage Alzheimer's patients have also found memory training very helpful, according to research conducted in 2002 by Dr Linda Clare from University College London.

It's believed that links in the brain's language-controlling areas can be gradually re-established through these games. Other studies have found that it is the variety of leisure and physical activities rather than the frequency or intensity which is more important. According to Dr. Glenn E. Smith of the Mayo College of Medicine, "if we engage both physical activity and cognitive stimulation, including these brain training games in a population-wide level, we have the potential to see fewer numbers of dementia in the population at large."

You can find more information on the website of The Lancet: www.thelancet.com.

Anti-Dementia Drugs

There are now drugs available which can help slow down progression and improve on symptoms, though as yet no drug can fully cure the condition. There are two main types of anti-dementia drugs that are used for people with Alzheimer's. As with other forms of treatment, evidence suggests that these medications are more likely to have a positive effect if they are taken in the early stages of the disease.

AChEI (Acetylcholinesterase Inhibitors)

According to research, nerve cells that use a chemical messenger called acetylcholine are found in lower numbers in the brains of those with Alzheimer's disease. Patients experience more severe symptoms as more nerve cells are lost. Increasing concentration of acetylcholine leads to increased communication between the nerve cells which use acetylcholine as a chemical messenger, which in turn can improve or stabilise symptoms.

AChEI is designed to prevent the enzyme acetylcholinesterase from breaking down the brain's supply of acetylcholine. There are three brands of acetylcholinesterase inhibitors:

"if we engage both physical activity and cognitive stimulation, including these brain training games in a population-wide level, we have the potential to see fewer numbers of dementia in the population at large."

Dr. Glenn E. Smith, Mayo College of Medicine

- Donepezil Hydrochloride (Aricept).
- Galantamine (Reminyl).
- Rivastigmine (Exelon).

At present in the UK, they are only licensed for use by people with mild to moderate Alzheimer's, although several studies have found that they do improve the symptoms of people with severe Alzheimer's. Taking this type of drug tends to benefit between 40% and 60% of people with Alzheimer's.

Improved thinking, memory, motivation and confidence, as well as reduced anxiety, have all been reported by people with Alzheimer's who have taken this medication (according to an Alzheimer's Society survey of 4,000 people).

Donepezil Hydrochloride

The first Alzheimer's drug to be licensed in the UK was Aricept (donepezil hydrochloride), manufactured by a company called Eisai. People tend to find that it improves their condition or at least stabilise it. This drug has been found by some studies to improve cognition and function, and reduce behavioural problems and hallucinations.

Everyone reacts differently to different medications, and it's important to note that Aricept does come with some potential side effects. These can include difficulty sleeping, lack of energy, stomach cramps, nausea, loss of appetite, headaches, diarrhoea and vomiting.

Rivastigmine

Made by Novartis Pharmaceutical, rivastigmine (Exelon) was the second Alzheimer's drug to be licensed in the UK. A positive effect on cognition has been identified by some studies. According to one of these studies, Alzheimer's patients who had high blood pressure found the drug more effective than those with normal blood pressure.

Most of the side effects associated with this drug will settle down over time, but when patients begin taking this drug they can experience vomiting, weight loss, loss of appetite and nausea. It's best to take this medication with a meal to avoid these side effects.

Galantamine

The third drug to be licensed in the UK was galantamine (Reminyl), which is made from the bulbs of narcissi and snowdrops. Research has found that Reminyl is effective in maintaining cognition and that it improves behaviour and functional ability. Launched in September 2000, this medication was co-developed by the Janssen Research Foundation and Shire Pharmaceuticals.

As with rivastigmine, the side effects associated with Reminyl usually settle down in time, but those taking it can initially experience vomiting and nausea. Sleeplessness, diarrhoea, loss of appetite, headache, tiredness, sleepiness, dizziness, weight loss and indigestions are also potential side effects.

Memantine (Ebixa)

One drug that works differently from the AChEI medications is Ebixa. Launched in October 2002, it is the first drug to be licensed for treatment in people with moderate to severe Alzheimer's. Because the other drugs are for people in the mild to moderate stages of the disease, they are likely to have been stopped before Ebixa is started. This drug works on the principle that when brain cells are damaged by Alzheimer's, the neurotransmitter glutamate is released in excessive quantities.

Glutamate is involved in normal memory and learning processes. Ebixa works to block this neurotransmitter. It protects the brain from cell regenerations by blocking the release of excess glutamate. Studies have also found that patients who take Ebixa experience significant benefits in memory, language and the ability to perform daily activities.

However, the NHS does not routinely prescribe this drug as it's believed that it isn't cost-effective as its benefits are too small. Further research on Ebixa has been recommended by NICE (the National Institute for Health and Clinical Excellence). Combining Aricept and Ebixa has been found to be more effective than using the drugs on their own, according to research conducted in the US.

In those in the mid- to later stages of Alzheimer's disease, Ebixa has been found to help with irritation and aggression, can improve everyday functions and slow down the progression of other symptoms. That said, some patients who have taken the drugs have experienced no benefits, so the effect really depends on the individual case.

Ebixa is not recommended for people with severe kidney problems because this group have not been tested. Once again, any potential side effects are likely to settle down over time. Those who have just started taking the drug may experience headaches, high blood pressure, fatigue and dizziness. We should also note that none of the medications mentioned above have been found to be addictive.

Other Medications

There is as likely a chance, if not more of a chance, of being on other medication, so it is worth finding out about other drugs. The drugs listed above are all that is currently available in the UK to deal directly with Alzheimer's disease. However, there are other drugs which can be used to treat specific symptoms of the disease.

We must note here that the following drugs can be prescribed for certain symptoms, but are not universally used by everyone who has Alzheimer's. Remember to always get professional medical advice from your GP. It is certainly a good idea to understand what they are and what they are used for as they may become an option at some point, but keep in mind that having Alzheimer's does not mean you'll need to take these medications.

Antipsychotics or Neuroleptics

People with dementia are often treated with antipsychotics and neuroleptics to help with restlessness, aggression and psychotic symptoms. Commonly used drugs in this category include trazodone, quetiapine and haloperidol. Many people in the more severe stages of the disease – around 60% of nursing home patients – take these medications. In the long term, the benefits are limited. Clinical trials have found that these drugs can reduce aggression and help with psychotic symptoms to a certain extent in the short term. The anti-dementia drug memantine may also be effective in treating aggression and other symptoms of agitation.

Antidepressants and Anticonvulsants

To reduce aggression and treat seizures, some people with Alzheimer's disease are given antidepressants like citalopram and trazodone, or anticonvulsants like carbamazepine and sodium valproate.

Many Alzheimer's sufferers struggle with depression. Coming to terms with the disease can be difficult, and depression in the early stages is often due to a reaction to the diagnosis itself. Later on, depression can also occur as a result of the brain's reduced chemical transmitters.

Alternative Medicine

In the hopes of being able to treat the disease with fewer side effects, many people look to natural and alternative medicine to treat Alzheimer's – as they do with any other illness. While some options have more evidence to support them than others, Alzheimer's is no different than any other condition so there are a few foods and natural products which are said to relieve symptoms.

Ginkgo Biloba

Long believed to enhance memory, ginkgo biloba is derived from the maidenhair tree. It is thought that ginkgo biloba increases blood flow to the brain. At present, it's estimated that more than 10% of people with dementia will try this herb at some point in their treatment. The research is uncertain on ginkgo biloba and whether it works for relieving Alzheimer's symptoms.

Some studies have suggested that the herb, which also acts as an antioxidant, could be almost as effective as AChEI medications. Others have reported improvements in social behaviour, understanding, dressing and eating.

More recently, a study published by the Alzheimer's Society in 2008 suggested that taking the herb could be a waste of time. This study found that ginkgo biloba did not prevent symptoms from getting worse and had no significant impact on the quality of life or mental function of those with Alzheimer's. One study into the effectiveness of the herb may have found a link between ginkgo biloba and a higher risk of stroke, but ethical considerations have so far prevented further research into this issue.

Few side effects have been pinned down entirely, but the herb has been found to delay blood clotting and should be avoided by those taking anticoagulants or those with bleeding disorders.

Vitamin E

Nuts, soybeans, corn, fish liver oils, whole-grain foods and sunflower seeds all contain Vitamin E. Recent studies have found that this chemical could be helpful in slowing down the development of Alzheimer's. It can, however, interfere with blood clotting and should not be consumed in large doses. Some experts recommend no more than two units a day.

One such study, published by the American Medical Association and reported in the Archives of Neurology, found that people aged 65 to 102 who ate fish at least once per week for three or more years experienced 35% less cognitive decline than those who ate less fish.

A more recent study found that those who took a vitamin E supplement (an oral dose of 1,000 international units (IU) of alpha tocopherol twice a day) declined more slowly in their ability to perform daily tasks than a control group who were given no supplements.

Balm Mint

Also known as lemon balm, this has been used as a sedative for some time. Several small studies have also found that lemon balm improves memory and appears to increase the activity of the chemical messenger acetylcholine. Sleep disorders, anxiety and stress are all said to benefit from its use.

This herb should not be used by those with diabetes or thyroid disease. It can cause too much drowsiness when combined with medications around surgery, so it should not be used for at least 2 weeks before any scheduled surgery.

Several small studies have also found that lemon balm improves memory and appears to increase the activity of the chemical messenger acetylcholine.

Other Treatments

Many of these are based on changing behaviours. Especially in the early stages, there are lots of treatments available that don't involve drugs.

Reality Orientation

Orientation and interaction with others can both be improved through reality orientation therapy, which involves continually telling or showing certain reminders to people with mild to moderate memory loss. Every conversation should include the time of day, day of the week and mention of familiar objects and people.

This therapy works best if it's performed in the home, with the individual surrounded by plenty of familiar objects. A psychotherapist can teach the method to the individual's caregivers or family.

Art Therapy

A significant improvement in Alzheimer's symptoms can be achieved through a 10-week art therapy course, according to research conducted at the University of Sussex and Goldsmiths College, London. Other research has backed this theory up and it certainly fits in with the advice to keep active. Participants found that their depression scores reduced, and they became more relaxed and sociable.

Summing Up

- Early-stages treatment for Alzheimer's can involve drugs, but won't always.

- Many anti-dementia drugs are most successful when taken early in the disease's progression.

- Research is constantly discovering new ways of dealing with the disease, and there's some evidence that alternative medicines can be effective.

- Most of all, keeping fit and active will go a long way to slowing down the progression of the disease.

- There are also several drugs on hand for the various symptoms.

- There are several anti-dementia drugs out there, so if one doesn't suit you it is likely that another will.

5

Why Is This Happening to Me?

I t's a question you're likely to ask. When you are first diagnosed with Alzheimer's, lots of thoughts go round in your head as you try to make sense of the situation. Did I do something to bring this on? What did I do to deserve this? Why did it have to be me? How could I have avoided this?

Have I Done Something to Cause It?

Did some aspect of your lifestyle cause this disease, or make you more prone to it? Did you do something wrong? When you're first diagnosed, it's easy to start looking back at your life and wondering if you brought this on yourself. The whole world is keen to find out what causes it so steps can be taken to prevent it. The truth is, of the most common types of dementia, Alzheimer's is probably one of the hardest for which to pin down a cause.

And in some respects, the constant research results being published in the national press isn't exactly helping things. Every month, another potential cause is theorised, with the underlying message suggesting that if these people hadn't done such-and-such a thing, they wouldn't have ended up this way. The most obvious thing you've done is get older – obviously something none of us can help.

What these reports are missing is perspective. The cure might be found in 20 years time, or it might be found next week. When we finally find out what that cure is, all of the research carried out over the last few decades will likely have been small contributing factors, steering the successful study in the right direction (or at least steering it away from dead ends).

For now, we know relatively little about what causes Alzheimer's, but we do know that vascular dementia has been linked to high blood pressure, high cholesterol, diabetes, heart problems and diet, and that Korsakoff's is strongly linked to excessive alcohol consumption. From what we have learnt so far and from research conducted on other forms of dementia and conditions affecting the brain, it is likely that lifestyle and environmental factors play a big part. A connection has also been made with previous head injuries.

We know that there are an estimated 15,000 people in the UK who have Alzheimer's at a relatively young age (under 65), but that your chances of developing Alzheimer's increase as you get older. Some experts have suggested that you should eat a healthy diet rich in omega 3 fatty acids, and try to keep the brain active by doing crosswords and other puzzles.

We know relatively little about what causes Alzheimer's, but we do know that vascular dementia has been linked to high blood pressure, high cholesterol, diabetes, heart problems and diet, and that Korsakoff's is strongly linked to excessive alcohol consumption.

Is it My Fault for Doing _____?

There are several theories and possible causes that have now been ruled out. It is a well studied area but a conclusive link has yet to be found. It seems as if there must be an explanation out there and that something we have done in the past must have caused it. Many people with Alzheimer's feel compelled to search for an explanation for developing the condition – it's probably the biggest negative result of the almost weekly news of research into causes of the condition.

Try to keep in mind that until we figure out the definite cause for the condition, focusing on it won't get you anywhere and isn't a constructive pastime. We know how difficult it can be to try and make yourself stop thinking about something.

Some studies have found higher than average levels of aluminium in the brains of people with Alzheimer's but other studies have found no link. For years, aluminium was topped as being a possible cause of Alzheimer's, and it's still a common misconception to this day. A direct link has yet to be found, despite numerous pieces of research and more than 40 years of theorising.

The Times released a story in 2006 about a 58-year-old woman who was exposed to high levels of aluminium for nearly 20 years, before dying from a rare form of Alzheimer's. However, this is more aluminium than the average person will ever be exposed to – 20 tonnes of aluminium sulphate had been dumped into her local water supply – so it hardly accounts for the high numbers of people all over the UK who develop Alzheimer's.

The development of Alzheimer's has also been widely blamed on high cholesterol, and many people have tried to prevent it by taking cholesterol-lowering drugs. However, the research done on this all contradicts each other, and no clear link has been determined.

We should note, however, that poor diet is one of the main causes of high cholesterol. It could be this rather than cholesterol which is to blame, as diet is one of the stronger links scientists have investigated in recent years.

What Part Do Family Genes Play?

If one of your parents had Alzheimer's, it is most likely that their illness was caused by a variety of lifestyle and environmental factors. Like many conditions, you can inherit genes which make you more susceptible to Alzheimer's but this does not necessarily mean you will develop it. To a certain extent, the impact of family genetics on your risk of developing Alzheimer's has been overstated.

With this first baby born free of the breast cancer gene in 2009, and an increasing interest in home DNA test companies like 23andMe and FamilyTree, the role of genetics in disease development has never been so widely discussed. We're becoming increasingly aware of what we can and can't prevent. Only 5% of Alzheimer's cases are diagnosed in those aged 30 to 60 and it is in a certain type of early-onset Alzheimer's called familial AD that the genetic aspect comes in.

There is a gene which increases your risk of late-onset Alzheimer's but it must be noted that this is just an increase and is not a certainty. For many people, if one of their parents had a condition like Alzheimer's, they feel like it's only a matter of time before they develop it themselves. Alzheimer's isn't that simple, though, and neither are many of the other "hereditary" conditions we hear about.

A person will have a high chance of developing Alzheimer's if they inherit even one of the mutant genes of familial AD from a parent, but this is still relatively unlikely as familial AD is not common. There are several genes involved in the development of Alzheimer's, some of which we still know little about. We really need to carry out more research into this area so we can put harmful misconceptions to rest.

The fact that genetics plays only a tiny role in your likelihood of developing Alzheimer's means that it's really not something worth worrying about. Energy should be put into what you can change, not what you can't. While there may be a slight increase in your likelihood of developing the condition if your parents had it, it's more worthwhile to spend a bit of time doing brainteasers and keeping yourself mentally active than to undertake expensive and unnecessary DNA testing.

Alzheimer's Research: What Causes It?

The amount of research studies and findings can be baffling, with different studies saying different things. It's really important that further research into Alzheimer's is carried out – this is something that will be repeated throughout this book. Many people feel that not enough money is spent on research when we take into consideration the number of people living with the disease and its growing prevalence in the population.

So just how close are we to finding causes and a cure? What have we achieved so far?

Researchers have been able to pin down some of the factors which can increase a person's risk of developing Alzheimer's, though no direct cause has been found yet. This increased risk is found in people who have high blood pressure, high cholesterol, or who smoke. It is also likely that keeping the brain active could help prevent onset.

This means that it is likely that the answer to what is the cause possibly lies at least partly in our lifestyle, even if we can't currently acknowledge anything as a direct cause.

A person's chance of developing dementia, according to one study conducted in New York in 2003, could be greatly reduced by doing a crossword puzzle at least four times a week. This has been taken on board by companies such as Nintendo whose Nintendo DI, previously marketed mainly at children, is now also being marketed at older people with the launch of its Brain Age game and with TV adverts showing this age group enjoying the game. Notably, while games specifically designed for 'brain training' can be a tempting buy as they're somewhat flashier than a £1 book of puzzles and more respectable than video games aimed at children and young people, a 2016 study carried out in the US found that these games had no real effect – or at least no greater effect than any other type of video game.

While no direct cause has been found as yet, it is generally accepted that a healthy lifestyle is the best way at present of preventing the disease. One Swedish study found that regular exercise can halve a person's chance of developing the disease. Several research studies have also confirmed a connection between an increased likelihood of developing Alzheimer's and a lack of regular physical exercise, showing us that a fit and active brain really needs a fit and active body to thrive.

Overweight people are 70% more likely to develop Alzheimer's, according to another study published in the British Medical Journal. So why does exercise make such a difference? Some suggest that exercise increases the blood flow to the brain, prolonging its health by keeping it active. So whether you're making sure your brain gets plenty of blood through exercise, doing your crosswords and other puzzles, or eating oily fish and other healthy foods to nourish the brain, the answer appears to lie in keeping your brain healthy through activity.

Coming to Terms with It

Acceptance can allow you to start talking positively with support workers, to take steps to join support groups, to make friends with others in the same situation and perhaps to help each other. At first you may decide to fight it and to not change your life, but you will eventually find that this is not possible and may end up making everything more upsetting.

Others may view it negatively and may go through a period of depression. Acceptance can allow you to move on a stage, to plan for the future and to make the necessary changes. But how do you come to terms with the fact that you have been diagnosed with a disease that has no cure and which will only get worse over time? A big part of accepting the diagnosis will always involve dealing with the "why me?" dilemma.

Everyone is different. Everyone has their own way of coping, and it'll never be easy. How early you are diagnosed and how quickly the disease progresses will have a big impact on how you come to terms with your condition. You'll have more time to come to terms with the disease if you're diagnosed early on, and you'll have more time to make plans for the later stages.

Finding out that there's a medical reason for the changes that are happening, and learning that it's not something like cancer or a brain tumour, can actually mean that being diagnosed with Alzheimer's is a relief for some people.

Each individual and their situation will determine how long it takes to accept what is happening. When you accept your disease, it'll become easier to accept support from those around you – whether that's practical or emotional.

Relatives can often take some time to come to terms with the fact that an Alzheimer's diagnosis has been made. It is not unusual for the relatives of people in the later stages of Alzheimer's to still be in a state of denial. Acceptance is often more challenging for the family than for the person who has the disease, though this may sound strange. It can go on for some time, as they attempt to search for an alternative diagnosis, or deny that the condition could possibly be real.

Summing Up

- It's completely normal to want to know how this has happened, and why it's happened to you. "Why me?" is a question that all patients will ask at some point or another.

- Differences exist between early-onset and late-onset dementia. While genetics and family links play a small role in the development of Alzheimer's, it's not as clear cut as the colour of your hair or eyes.

- Every research study which is carried out takes us one step closer, even if we don't have the answers just yet.

- It's normal to feel shocked or to be in denial about your condition at first, but it is necessary to accept your condition if you want to make plans and take action.

- Family often find it harder to come to terms with the situation and this may continue long term.

- Looking for a cause and a reason may be the first step in accepting Alzheimer's.

- Research is constantly going on into causes and cures.

- Due to the nature of the illness, it is harder to pin down the causes of Alzheimer's, with more being known about other forms of dementia.

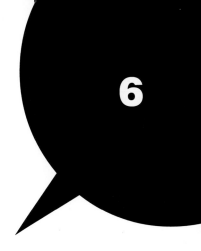

6

What Do I Do Now?

You may feel that you should be doing something, making changes to your life and preparing for the future but when, and where, do you start? Many people have spent months, sometimes years, trying to get a diagnosis. The time following diagnosis can seem a bit empty, especially if you've been waiting for your diagnosis for a long time. It's hard to know what to do next when the thing you've been working toward is finally achieved.

What You Should Do

Take some time to get used to the idea, to read up on Alzheimer's and to think about what you want and where you feel you need to make changes. There really isn't any rush to do anything. Where partners or other family members have been at a loss to explain the strange behaviour, diagnosis can bring a new level of understanding. They should be able to provide you with support, both emotionally and physically, when required.

Steps can be taken to slow progression and drugs can be prescribed to do this. Nowadays, people are diagnosed much earlier on and often keep on working and living a normal life. Earlier diagnosis is better – this is one thing that all experts can agree on. An early diagnosis allows for more effective treatment, but it can also put minds at rest, especially if the cause of the symptoms has really been worrying you.

You can finally focus on the true cause once other potential conditions have been ruled out. It used to be the case that symptoms had to be really obvious and having a severe impact on a person's life before a diagnosis was made. By the time a doctor said it was Alzheimer's, it was more a confirmation of what everyone knew than a new piece of information.

Terry Pratchett didn't have to stop writing when he was diagnosed with Alzheimer's, and you don't need to stop doing what you love, either.

Life doesn't end once you have been diagnosed! More likely than not, there will be plenty of time for you to make preparations and adjust to your diagnosis. But even if you have decided to do things on your own, at some stage friends and family will need to be told.

Telling family and friends should be at the top of your to-do list. As you went through visits to specialists and various medical tests, it's likely that your friends were there to give you support.

The early stage of the disease is the time when medication is most effective. Speaking to your specialist or family doctor about medication is another important thing to do after diagnosis. There are several drugs available – talk to your GP or specialist to find out which one suits you best. The earlier you do this, the more time you'll have to try and change medications and figure out which works for you. Find out what options you have and take all the time you need to decide which medication you want to take – if any.

Nutrition and what you eat is also worth considering if you haven't done so already. A good, regular diet from the different food groups is recommended. It's advisable to optimise nutrient intake at this stage, as weight loss in the middle and late stages of Alzheimer's is very common.

A healthy all-round approach should be taken to your diet right now, with a focus on preventing anaemia and any vitamin deficiency. Research has explored the benefits of different food types in preventing Alzheimer's, but right now your goal should just be to eat healthily.

As explained earlier, there is much evidence that keeping the mind active is good for slowing down the onset of the disease which is why it is a good idea to take up a new interest. Don't immediately rule out going to the places you usually go to or holidaying in places you have always dreamt of visiting. You can help avoid depression and insomnia if you take care to stay active and keep doing the things you love.

Now is the time to do all the things you've been putting off for years. Consider looking into taking up a hobby which will keep your mind active and occupy your time (if you don't already have one!), whether that's watching films, visiting museums and the theatre, or making art.

Plan ahead and tell those close to you of your wishes. The final thing you need to do is think about what you want in the future. You might not always be able to drive, so make plans for what you'll do instead. Somewhere down the line, you'll also need to decide who you trust to look after your affairs, so speak to someone today about who should have your power of attorney.

Somewhere down the line, you'll also need to decide who you trust to look after your affairs, so speak to someone today about who should have your power of attorney.

What Changes Should I Make?

Keep a bit of routine. Plan your day so that you are not rushed and allow yourself more time than you would have done previously. Through time you will find that you have good days and bad days, as well as times of the day when you are not doing so well. Decide what doesn't need to be done immediately and plan to do it another day when you are feeling more able.

Aim to do difficult tasks at a time of day when you tend to feel best. If you need help with the housework, arrange for this. Speak to friends and neighbours who may be able to recommend someone. If it'll allow you to manage on your own for longer and have a better quality of life, it's vital that you become comfortable with asking for help. This can be tricky as many of us value our independence and want to preserve it for as long as we can.

You should look into companies and individuals who can help you if your family aren't available to do so. Many of your bills can be paid by direct debit, and this is something worth setting up. It'll reduce the number of occasions where you may have problems handling money, and will save you the effort of having to go to the bank or post office to pay them yourself.

Try to accept that everyone struggles sometimes. Everyone has bad days when they're less capable of doing what needs to be done, so postpone things that can be done later and ask for help with any urgent matters.

Don't let anyone hurry you. If there's a task that you need to (or want to) finish, finish it in your own time.

Make sure that you have a reason to get up each day and go out as often as possible – you can do this by arranging activities and meetings regularly.

Changes which May Help with the Disease

A 2009 study conducted at the Mayo Clinic in the USA suggested that activities such as reading, playing games, using a computer and doing craft activities can reduce the risk of memory loss. Try to keep in mind that although many elderly people have taken to buying the Nintendo DS and similar devices to play and stave off dementia, this has been found to be no more effective than cheaper alternatives like newspaper crosswords. Games consoles can be a fun way to keep the brain active and pass your time so there's nothing wrong with buying one if you fancy it, just don't let misinformation cheat you into spending more money than you need to.

Arrange for a friend or family member to remind you of any appointments you have. Many people find that triggers work. There are many things you can do to help trigger your memory as remembering things gets more challenging. For example, you could keep a list of the phone numbers you use most often beside your telephone so you can access them easily if you forget them.

Try picking up a small date-per-page calendar that you have to change at the start of each day, as this may help you keep track of the date.

Consider visiting a day centre on a regular basis. They will organise stimulating projects, help you with memory exercises and may organise days out to local attractions. Most day centres will pick you up and drop you off so you don't need to worry about getting there and back. Make sure you still go out often and that you don't begin to become isolated.

Find out where your nearest day centre is, and what else is available in your area. Day centres have lots of great benefits, such as providing you with social activities with others in the same position, and helping you get into a routine.

Some Things Aren't Worth Worrying About

The more you think about things, the worse a situation can seem. After a while you will get used to the ups and downs, and will learn to adjust your life to suit. Many of your worries will be unfounded and will just make you more stressed. Speak to people about your concerns and ensure that your mind is put at rest. You may well end up worrying about worrying if you let your worrying get too bad. Try to cut it out early!

Most people will be only too pleased to help. Asking for help from family and friends, or asking to spend time with those you love, are not things you should worry about. Those who really care about you will be happy to help, so try not to feel guilty.

Some days are worse than others, but don't worry about that. There's every likelihood that tomorrow will be much better than today.

Worrying can lead to depression if it's allowed to go on for too long. It's just not worth it, as worrying doesn't change anything. Speak to people about any worries you have, and avoid keeping things to yourself.

Who Can Help?

Sometimes you have to make the first move and ask for help. While you can access professional help, emotional and practical support from the people who care about you cannot be replaced. They know you and hopefully at times will offer help without you needing to ask. Your first port of call should be your family and friends, even though there are a number of other places you can go to for help.

Family and friends can offer you long-term support that you just won't get anywhere else. Some of the people who care about you won't know if they should offer help or not, as they'll be worried about offending you. Others will offer support straight away. Whether they come forward without prompting or not, you'll likely find that the people who love you have just been waiting for an excuse to help you.

Which Organisations Can Help?

If you want to access services, your local authority is a good place to start. They will tell you what services and help you are due. It's best to do some research and find out what applies to your local area, but in many parts of the country the department you need will be called Direct Care Services. If you require it, some local authorities can even organise a cleaner for you.

The Alzheimer's Society and Alzheimer's Scotland can also provide support and advice, and are excellent points of reference for the times when you don't know who to turn to and don't know what services you can access. They'll be able to explain which services can help you, and put you in touch with them if necessary. Memory clinics can also provide treatment for people with Alzheimer's. The Glasgow Memory Clinic was established in 2000 and is now based within a purpose built facility at the West of Scotland Science Park, Bearsden, Glasgow.

The government announced plans for memory clinics in every UK town in 2008. While this may not have happened quite yet, services have been improving. According to the Dementia Statistics Hub, the number of people seen by memory services rose 31% from 2013 to 2014, with the number of identified memory services rising from 214 to 222.

These numbers have really increased over the last 20 years, though memory clinics have been around since the late 1980s. The NHS website (www.nhs.uk) is a great place to start. They have information on all the clinics in the UK, as well as a good page that specifically deals with dementia, the services available to you, and advice for people with the condition (www.nhs.uk/conditions/dementia/). Some memory clinics are based in hospital, so it's worth checking to see if your local hospital has a service like this.

Dementia helplines, some of which offer a 24-hour service, are available in various parts of the country. Both the Alzheimer's Society and Alzheimer's Scotland run dementia helplines, as do organisations such as For Dementia, whose helpline is manned by Admiral Nurses. When all you need is someone to talk to, these can give you all the support you need.

The government announced plans for memory clinics in every UK town in 2008. While this may not have happened quite yet, services have been improving.

Summing Up

- Following your diagnosis, you should spend some time thinking about what you want for the future. There's no real rush to take action right away.

- Try your best to stay physically and mentally active.

- Life can get easier if you make some small changes to your routine.

- Allowing yourself to worry will only result in you getting upset, and won't help anything.

- There are lots of organisations that you can turn to if you need them, but your friends and family should also try to help.

- The Alzheimer's Society and Alzheimer's Scotland are two of the best places to start.

- Speak to people about any concerns you have.

- Don't be afraid to ask for help.

- Keep up an interest in life and living.

- The first people you should tell are friends and family.

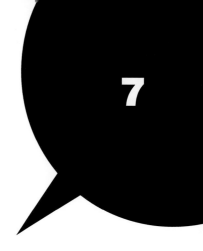

7

Friends and Family

With any luck, your family and friends will have been supporting you since day one. A friend or family member may have been with you when you received a diagnosis. However, for some people, family and friends will not know about the problems that have been happening. If anyone knows about your condition, consider asking them for advice about what and how you should tell the people you love.

When Should I Tell My Family and Friends?

This question has no one right answer. These are the people who will be around as your condition progresses and to whom the term "Alzheimer's" will have more meaning. Even if you have had your suspicions, it may well still come as a shock and it may take you a bit of time to accept. Sometimes it is the people closest to us who are the hardest to tell and they can take the news badly.

Sometimes family and friends are the ones to notice changes first, or to at least voice their concerns. If those close to you already know, it could be an idea for them to tell others for you. Ideally, the subject will have already come up when talking about what could be causing your symptoms, and those closest to you will already know that you've been going to specialists for tests.

Ideally, they will have been the ones preparing you for this outcome and supporting you, not the other way around. Not everyone has these ideal situations, though, and how close you are with your family and the strength of your relationship will likely have determined how much those around you know about your condition. Be prepared for the fact that you may be hit by a variety of reactions when you tell people.

Your family are likely to be the people who have the strongest reaction, and feel the diagnosis the most. People can be surprising – you may find that once you start telling people, life becomes easier as you start being offered more support. Before you begin telling anyone else, you may decide that you need to take some time for yourself to get used to the diagnosis before dealing with anyone else's feelings. It allows you to get used to the idea and to prepare for other people's reactions and questions.

Once they have had some time to themselves to adjust, a lot of people find that they're better equipped to break the news to their family and friends. Try not to spend too much time fretting about telling people.

At the end of the day, it's your decision when you want to tell people.

When you were first given the diagnosis, how did you feel? You're likely to have felt a wide range of emotions. Other people are likely to feel a similar mixture of emotions, and you may have to wait for the news to sink in a little.

What to Tell Them and How

"I have Alzheimer's" does cover all bases and to a certain extent it is best to get straight to the point. This may seem obvious at first. Choose a time when people are not too busy. Don't be too surprised if people ask what you think are stupid questions. Others may simply be keen to find out more and may unfortunately be voicing their opinions in the wrong way.

Whatever you say, though, this is big news and is likely to set in motion lots of separate discussions, either over time or straight away. Many people have little knowledge of the disease and will feel that they owe it to you to find out more. They may want to ask you questions at a later date – remember that you have probably had a bit of time to get used to the idea, so others will need this too.

Ensure that the person you are telling has time to listen. You might end up walking away with the incorrect impression that the person doesn't care if you tell them while they're busy or distracted, as they will not have properly processed what you told them. After telling the first few people, you may find that things get easier and that you have the answers ready.

Some of the stigma around conditions like Alzheimer's disease still lingers, even though we've come a long way since the old-fashioned, incorrect ideas and opinions of the past. People sometimes say silly things they don't really mean without thinking, so try to be patient. Allowing people time to get used to the idea before having a more detailed, face-to-face discussion can be handy, so some people prefer to spread the news by telephone.

Questions tend to snowball once one or two have been asked and answered, so be prepared to deal with lots of questions once the news has sunk in. You might not have the answers to all of the questions your friends and family have, but sometimes pointing people in the direction of a good information source can be even better than a direct answer.

People can surprise you, positively or negatively. Make sure you're emotionally prepared before taking on this sort of discussion.

Talking to Young Children about Alzheimer's

Whether you tell the children in your family or not depends very much on their age and maturity level. The children's parents should judge each situation as it arises. If you are regularly making mistakes, it is likely that children will notice and comment on it. In many cases, you will not need to tell the young children in your family about your condition – children can be very accepting of people's behaviour. They're more likely to just think their grandparent is pretending or being silly on purpose, and may laugh at the "sillier" things you do.

Remember that a child's parent may well tell them about your condition if you don't do it yourself. In this case, hopefully the parent will take into account the needs of both you and the child before deciding how much needs to be said. But at the same time, if the person with Alzheimer's begins to get aggressive or show signs of unacceptable behaviour, they should remove the child.

Whether you tell the children in your family or not depends very much on their age and maturity level. The children's parents should judge each situation as it arises.

It's a good idea to encourage a strong relationship between young children and older people, as it can be beneficial for both parties (especially the elderly person).

Who to Tell Outside the Family

Do you really need to tell other people? Other than family and friends, should you be telling anyone else about your condition?

You may also want to tell people who see you regularly – acquaintances rather than friends. Only tell who you want to and who you feel needs to know. Outside of your close friends and family, it's not worth spending time worrying about telling people – this really isn't a priority right now. Tell your neighbours if you're on friendly terms and feel it would be helpful.

A neighbour may offer to start looking in on you or to do shopping for you. It may be good for them to know in case you have an accident or need help when none of your family and friends are available. You may also find comfort confiding in people at church, if you regularly attend one.

How to Deal with People's Responses

Everyone acts differently in response to this sort of news, so it's likely that you'll be met with a variety of reactions. Practical and emotional support may be offered by some of the people you tell, as they'll be trying to act supportive. When you are upset or have concerns, these people may provide an extra ear to listen.

It is great to receive immediate support from loved ones, but don't be too disheartened if some people don't react the way you expect. Some people can respond in a more negative, dismissive manner if they don't believe you're showing the symptoms they've heard of, or don't believe the disease exists. They may question the doctor's diagnosis and may tell you that they think the specialist is wrong.

They may not categorise your symptoms as being those of someone with Alzheimer's as they may only be familiar with the symptoms of later-stage Alzheimer's.

In some cases, people might make no effort to show any support or display any real reaction, and it'll be difficult to tell if they've even taken in what you've said.

Try to be patient – it often takes time to process this type of news properly.

Coping with Negative Reactions

Coming to terms with Alzheimer's can be hard enough, but having to cope with other people's reactions can seem like a step too far. It can be very upsetting if your news is met with a negative reaction. Time may change their mind – but it may not. Some people find it difficult to cope with such things and may not have the strength of character to react well.

It can easily feel like your family and friends have let you down at a time when you need them the most. You can't change people's personalities and shouldn't try. Understanding why people react the way they do can make dealing with these interactions a little easier. The people who don't believe you can be a challenging obstacle to deal with.

If someone isn't informed about the disease, they may base their opinions on the limited portrayals they've seen in the media and won't know that there are different ways it can show itself. There are also the people with unrealistic expectations of miracle cures. Always remember that the initial reactions you are met with may just be temporary.

Increasing media coverage of Alzheimer's may hit them eventually or someone else with a sharp tongue may force them to alter their opinions. You shouldn't stress yourself out by trying to convince people you have a disease that you didn't want to have in the first place. This isn't your responsibility, and there probably isn't much you can do anyway.

A person may have their own personal reasons for reacting negatively if they're close to you in age. They might not know what to say or do and could say something inappropriate when they do try. Alzheimer's is a life-changing condition, and they may have just realised that it could easily have been them that developed the disease, not you.

Accepting that the person may not be available for you to confide in for now is likely the best you can do.

Some people won't know what to do to be supportive. They'll feel upset on your behalf, but might not know how to react. Try to understand that sometimes when people find themselves in difficult situations like this, they can easily say something they don't mean and will regret purely because they're scrambling for something, anything, to say.

Try to remember that the people around you care about you, and their way of showing that or staying positive might just be coming out all wrong.

Think about how long it took you to accept your Alzheimer's diagnosis. Friends and family need that time too. It's likely that you started getting used to the idea even before you were properly diagnosed. There's every chance that the people who didn't respond positively or even called you a liar will get used to it over the first year, and will be ready to support you when they've had time to think.

Case Study

"My friends and family had a mixed reaction to my diagnosis. Some didn't believe the diagnosis, and others just weren't interested. Maybe some of them chose not to believe because it was easier than actually processing the information.

"A small group of my friends were really understanding, and they continue to support me to this day. They offer me practical support, and ask me how I'm getting on. Some of the people who reacted poorly at first just took a while to come to terms with the news. They're really supportive now, especially my sister." – Craig, age 78.

Think about how long it took you to accept your Alzheimer's diagnosis. Friends and family need that time too.

Summing Up

- Telling the people you love that you've been diagnosed with Alzheimer's can be really difficult.

- Don't start the discussion when the person you're talking to is doing or thinking about something else. Choose your timing wisely.

- It's likely you'll be met with a mixture of reactions, and some may even respond very negatively.

- You may find that the people who react badly just need time to accept it. This is big news, and it can take people a while to get used to it.

- Negative reactions can be due to a number of factors and should not upset you.

- Be prepared for lots of questions. If you can't answer them, point friends and family in the direction of good sources of information.

- You may find that you need time to get used to the idea yourself before you tell others, or you may feel that they can provide the support you need at this time.

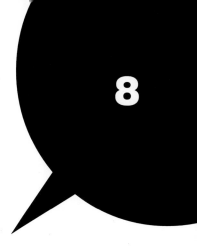

8

Making Plans

There are people you are legally obliged to tell such as the Driver and Vehicle Licensing Agency (DVLA) and insurance companies, but there are also legal steps you should take in order to make life easier later on. Your priority needs to be telling people close to you about your diagnosis. When they know about the situation, your friends and family will be able to help you to inform the relevant authorities and start planning for the future.

Sit down with someone you trust and discuss what needs to be done as soon as you feel ready.

Power of Attorney

Once you're ready, you'll need to make plans for the future. One of the first things you should do is decide who should have the power to look after your affairs when you're no longer able to. This can take a lot of pressure off you and your family as time moves on, and also means that you can make your wishes known now and trust they'll be taken into account later on.

Wales and England

A power of attorney is a legal document which allows you to nominate a person to look after your affairs on your behalf. A fee does apply for this. Ideally you should choose more than one person to avoid anyone abusing their power and they should be people who will work together. On 1st October 2007, lasting power of attorney (LPA) replaced enduring power of attorney.

There are two types of lasting power of attorney in England and Wales: a property and affairs LPA and a personal welfare LPA. It's often a good idea to talk to a solicitor before registering your new attorneys, but you aren't required to. When selecting your attorney, try to pick someone you trust to have your best interests at heart, and who looks after their own affairs and finances effectively.

A personal welfare LPA will make decisions on your health, any treatment you may be offered and on your welfare, for example where you live. Of course, they will be expected to listen to the advice of nurses, doctors and other healthcare specialists before making these decisions. Your property, money and other affairs will be looked after by your property and affairs LPA.

Your LPA form has to be registered at the Office of the Public Guardian for it to be legally recognised.

Scotland

As in Wales and England, the Scottish system also uses two types of power of attorneys: a welfare power of attorney and a continuing (financial) power of attorney. As in England, the form must be registered at the Office of the Public Guardian (Scotland). One power of attorney can be made to cover both aspects or two separate ones appointing different people.

A welfare power of attorney appoints someone to make decisions about medical and care issues and other personal matters, while a continuing power of attorney is responsible for looking after your property and money. If your first choice has to step down, a replacement attorney can also be appointed.

A solicitor is required to sign a certificate of capacity which must accompany your power of attorney form.

Northern Ireland

If you're based in Northern Ireland, you can register an Enduring Power of Attorney at any point provided you're over the age of 18 and deemed mentally capable of understanding the process.

All Enduring Powers of Attorney need to be registered with the High Court (Office of Care and Protection) before they can come into effect, but registration is not required until it's believed that you are no longer capable of managing your own affairs. An Enduring Power of Attorney will allow someone to gain control over your property and other affairs, but you can talk to your solicitor while setting this up to put a limit on their powers – for example, you may choose not to give someone the power to sell your house.

For more information about power of attorney in Northern Ireland, visit nidirect.gov.uk or talk to your solicitor.

Informing the DVLA

You are legally required to tell the DVLA if you've been diagnosed with dementia. Your car insurance may become invalid if you do not do so, and you may be fined up to £1,000. They will send you a questionnaire and will request a report from your GP. This doesn't necessarily mean that you won't be allowed to drive anymore, though! The DVLA will need to make an assessment, but if you're still in the early stages of the disease you may be able to continue driving for some time.

You can call the Authority for support of an Alzheimer's patient you care for is refusing to inform the DVLA. They won't get in trouble – the authority will just send out a standard form for them to fill in which will ask if they have anything they'd like to tell the DVLA about (such as dementia).

Informing Your Insurance Provider

People are often caught out because they fail to inform insurance companies of changes to their health or circumstances. Your motor insurance company should be told about your condition as early as possible, as we've already discussed. You should also highlight your Alzheimer's when filling out forms for new insurance policies. You risk invalidating your insurance if you don't inform them, as you may be breaking the clauses of your agreement.

You are legally required to tell the DVLA if you've been diagnosed with dementia. Your car insurance may become invalid if you do not do so, and you may be fined up to £1,000.

If you're in any doubt as to how to go about this, just give your provider a call.

Finding new insurance policies may involve a bit of shopping around – some companies don't accept applications from people with pre-existing medical conditions, but there are some companies out there who will cover you anyway.

Travelling with Alzheimer's

You will be able to judge for yourself what you feel able to do and how far you are able to go. Travelling and going away on holiday does not need to be taken off the table just because you've been diagnosed with Alzheimer's. Speak to the airline or travel company to see if they can offer assistance if you have any concerns.

Making Adaptations

The first thing you should look at is your attitude to assistance. If you have always been an independent person, asking for help can seem like giving up your independence or giving in to the condition. But if you feel things are getting on top of you, or if there are some jobs you just aren't able to do, then look around for help. You should view it as taking steps to prolong your independence.

There are some changes that are worth considering that aren't necessary, but can help to make life simpler and less overwhelming. Try to have a positive attitude to change. You'll be able to do a lot more on your own if you arrange a little additional support.

Whether you're asking a stranger how to use a public telephone or asking someone where the nearest bus stop is because it's slipped your mind for a second, most of the people you encounter will have no problem with being asked for help. They will assist, accept your thanks and move on, quickly forgetting. It's really unlikely that any of these people will give any thought to why you are asking, or bother to judge you for not knowing something.

Most people just don't have the time for that.

Paying by direct debit is becoming increasingly common and in many cases results in a discount. Consider arranging for your bills to be paid by direct debit if you don't already. This will mean you don't need to worry about handling money or going out to pay them in person, and will help you avoid forgetting to pay them by a certain date.

Employing a cleaner is another thing worth considering. Many people enjoy housework and if you're in that group, great! But if you do need help, you can get it by contacting your local authority or asking family or friends for a recommendation. You should be able to find someone who can visit regularly – even an hour or two a week can make a big difference!

If you've been thinking about moving somewhere to be closer to your family, now might be a good time to do it. Take a long term view of properties and find somewhere you will be happy living in for a long time. Ask someone you trust to help you organise your possessions and look for a suitable place. Moving into a new area and meeting new people can be very stressful and confusing in the later stages of the disease, so aim to move early so you have plenty of time to settle in.

Looking for Local Support

Once you start looking, you will be surprised at how much help there is out there. Friends you may make at a support group for people with Alzheimer's may be able to tell you what there is locally which can result in you discovering other services that your local authority provides. In most areas you will be able to find support, whether that is people to speak to, professional advice or practical support locally.

The help and support available to people in your situation is increasing as people become more aware of dementia. You'll find a list of organisations in the back of the book who will be able to help you, or at the very least put you in touch with someone who can. A postcode lottery still exists with regards to dementia services. Some areas are much better catered for than others, and unfortunately the level of support available is not the same throughout the country.

Many people find it easier to learn about other support options once they've started accessing one means of support.

Not all benefits are restricted to people on low incomes and some are not means tested. Carers may be able to claim Carer's Allowance if they care for someone for more than 35 hours a week. You may be due benefits you haven't heard about, so it's worth doing a little research if you're in need of financial support. You may find that a little extra money could make it possible to access services that make your life easier – such as a cleaner – even if you feel that you're managing alright as you are.

People over the age of 65 can access an Attendance Allowance, while those under 65 can get a Disability Living Allowance.

It's always worth finding out what you're due, even if you don't intend to access it right now.

Getting Ready for the Future

Appointing a power of attorney and settling personal affairs can leave you with a sense of relief that things have been taken care of and that decisions are now in the hands of someone trustworthy.

Take time to make an action plan, noting what you want to happen and any considerations that you want taken into account. If you haven't already done so, make a will. You should view it as your way of ensuring your wishes are followed. Organising power of attorney is one of the main steps you should take and it is certainly advisable to have everything in place long before it is needed.

You should begin to prepare for the future now, as your condition will worsen at some stage. It will allow you time to look into care arrangements and to decide about nursing homes. Getting ready early means you won't be rushed into making any snap decisions later on. It's less stressful to make preparations while you're still capable and have time to think properly about things.

Many nursing homes are accustomed to showing relatives around, and would be more than happy to let you have a look if you want to see for yourself. Nursing homes do admit that although they regularly show people around, in the vast majority of cases these people are relatives and carers and most people prefer not to think too much about reaching this stage.

A lot of people find the idea of choosing a care home upsetting, and that's alright. Talk to someone you trust, let them know your preferences, and trust that they'll make the right call in the future. Tell them what you do and don't want from a care home, and ask them to keep this in mind when the time comes.

Make sure you communicate your plans to the person or people you have given power of attorney, as well as anyone else you think should know.

Last, but definitely not least, make sure your affairs are in order so that they are easy to work with further down the line. Appointing a power of attorney and settling personal affairs can leave you with a sense of relief that things have been taken care of and that decisions are now in the hands of someone trustworthy. If you want to put any investments into trust, do it now.

This will make life easier for your family, and will save a lot of time and unnecessary expenses. It's understandable that some people prefer to put off thinking about these things, never mind writing down their wishes, writing wills and granting powers of attorney. These are big steps, and many aspects of them can be upsetting for some people.

Some people find it to be a positive experience, though, as they are able to be proactive and maintain control rather than just giving up. Some people find it very reassuring to know they have their affairs in order.

Summing Up

- There are people you are legally obliged to tell about your condition, other than your friends and family. There are also a number of things you can do that will relieve some of the pressure this condition can put on you.

- You are legally required to inform the DVLA of your diagnosis, though you may still be allowed to drive for some time.

- Ask for help whenever you need it. The majority of people will be more than happy to lend a hand.

- Set out an emergency action plan for when your condition worsens. Let the people you trust know what you want to happen.

- Look at what local support there is. While this varies throughout the country, through speaking to people in similar circumstances you will find out what is available.

- Make a list of insurance companies you need to inform – motor insurance should be top of that list.

- Appointing people with power of attorney should be done early on. A solicitor is not required in England and Wales but you may find that it is worth paying the money for one in order to receive some expert advice.

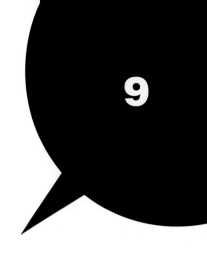

9

Living with Someone Suffering from Alzheimer's

The first indicators that someone has Alzheimer's are often spotted first by the people close to them. This chapter is addressed to the people who care – the wife, daughter, sibling, son, or husband of the person with Alzheimer's. It may be especially helpful to the partner, spouse or anyone else who lives in the same house as the person with Alzheimer's, the people living with the condition without actually having the condition.

How Do You React?

A diagnosis provides an explanation and a starting point for learning how to cope, but it can also bring a range of emotions including fear. You may feel angry that this has happened to someone you love, sadness at what you have lost or guilt at your lack of patience and anger when things are really bad. How are you meant to respond when you find out that the person you love has Alzheimer's disease?

What thoughts go through your head? What are you meant to do? It can seem like someone is slowly turning into a different person when they develop Alzheimer's. Sadly, marriages can sometimes deteriorate long before the diagnosis as partners struggle to understand why their loved one is acting so out of character. They may be at a loss for an explanation, or put it all down to work stress or even an affair.

We all married for particular reasons and were attracted to our partner for their characteristics. If it's your spouse who has the disease, it can feel like the person you married has disappeared and left behind someone who looks the same but acts completely differently. Unfamiliar, child-like qualities can gradually appear in the person you've been married to for years, and it's a weird thing to see.

At times you may feel that the stress is getting too much and that you are at the end of your tether. In many cases, couples express that their life would have been much easier if the diagnosis of Alzheimer's had been made sooner.

However, in other cases the diagnosis just brings in a fear of the future and of deterioration, to replace the existing fear of the unknown. Total exhaustion is also inevitable.

New negative emotions might creep in. Maybe you feel resentful about what you've lost, or bitter about having to cut back on other activities and commitments, or giving up work.

You're suddenly faced with new physical and mental burdens, and the work and care required from you can become very tiring.

You may no longer feel close to your partner as their behaviours become increasingly alien to you. If your partner was previously the care-giver in the relationship, becoming a carer can be particularly jarring. It can be helpful to see this as the beginning of a new relationship, rather than the end of an old one.

There will still be laughter and love, and having a good sense of humour can mean that you both see the funny side of things at times. All the negative emotions that you feel now don't mean that there won't be more positive ones down the line.

Supporting Your Partner

The most important way you can support your partner is by just being there and showing you care. Your partner will need you and your support more than any specialist, miracle cure or medication. This can seem like too much to cope with for some people, as the responsibility can appear overwhelming. There will be people you can turn to who can answer your questions, but when it is late at night and you are sitting alone thinking about things, a book can seem like a friend and can answer so many of your questions before you even ask them. This really will make it easier to cope.

Acceptance is vital for everyone. You'll have to start taking practical steps to help deal with the condition, but you can't do this until you've accepted the situation.

Try to get together as much information as you can.

Anything your partner does that's out of character can be explained if you gather information on their condition. There's so much information out there about why Alzheimer's sufferers act the way they do. It'll be easier not to get angry if you know that your partner no longer eats potatoes or cauliflower because their brain can't differentiate between them and the plate, than if you think they're just being picky. It also means you know to use coloured plates. Things can still be frustrating, but that frustration should become more manageable when it's not accompanied by confusion.

Psychiatric nurses who care for the same people for years are adamant that the person they have got to know in the later stages is still very much a person with their own personality. Try to view these changes in your partner as gaining another side to the person you love, rather than losing them forever. This is definitely still your partner, however different they may seem from the person they used to be.

Try and bring as much positive into your lives as possible. Setting aside some special time just to spend together can be helpful for many couples. Some people find it helpful to spend some of this time looking at a memory book that might include newspaper clippings about major events that happened in your life, and photographs from the different stages of your relationship. Why things get tough, try forgetting about tomorrow and just focussing on enjoying today. There's no reason that life can't still be fun.

Some people find it helpful to spend some of this time looking at a memory book that might include newspaper clippings about major events that happened in your life, and photographs from the different stages of your relationship.

Keeping an Eye Out

An occupational therapist will be able to advise you on things to look out for, changes to make and whether you are able to receive funding to make alterations to your home. It's a good idea to take steps sooner rather than later to reduce risks, as dementia increases the risk of accidents in the home.

Dangerous liquids such as bleach or paint should be kept safely away. You should call someone as soon as possible if any repairs are required in your house. Even if something doesn't seem like it could cause a problem, try looking at it with a view to the long term, and make changes if you think there's any chance it could cause an injury.

If you feel that your partner has started to forget where things are, then steps can easily be taken to help them, like labelling each cupboard in the kitchen. Be sure to be on the lookout for signs that your partner's condition is progressing, and be aware of any changes in their behaviour. They may start to forget how to do household tasks such as turning on the washing machine or find they are unable to use the telephone.

Try and take note if they seem to have difficulty knowing what time of day it is, and look for changes in their sleeping pattern (have they suddenly started taking naps?) Try and watch out for any sign that their long term memory is getting worse, even though the best known symptom of Alzheimer's is a loss of short term memory. Forgetting who they're married to is a bigger issue than forgetting they have an appointment with the hairdresser.

One of the most worrying symptoms you're likely to encounter is wandering. It's something that happens in many people with Alzheimer's, and they aren't always able to find their way home if they go too far. This is something you'll need to take steps to prevent if it becomes an issue with your partner. Even a simple set of windchimes at the front door can do the trick.

Various alarm systems are available which will let you know when your partner has opened the door to go out, and there are also tracking devices you can use to find them if they do go walkabouts.

Support Groups for Family

It is easy to let hobbies slide and give up on the activities you used to look forward to so much. It is important to remember that you are a person in your own right and have a separate identity to being a full time carer. Finding time for yourself is not something you should just consider – it is something you must do for yourself and your family. Aim to keep or regain some "me time" every week.

Many people find they forget to look after themselves because they've become so engrossed in looking after their loved one. Our health and behaviour can suffer as a result. You will be much better placed to care for your partner if you've had a bit of a break and some relief from the focus and pressure of caring for someone with Alzheimer's disease.

Keeping up a hobby will only take up your attention for a few hours a week, but having those few hours to yourself can be as beneficial as taking a trip away.

Go for a coffee with a friend, or take a walk in the park on your own. For many, relief comes in the form of talking and sharing problems and experiences. It doesn't have to be anything fancy or expensive, so long as it's something you want to be doing.

Don't refuse the offer if someone calls round out of the blue and offers to care for your partner for a couple of hours while you take a break.

Try to organise a visit to a support group and see if it suits you. Friends may give you advice, and it is good to talk to people you know and trust, but support groups provide that added extra because most people there have or have had a similar experience to you. Those who have been through (or are going through) the same thing are you are easily the best people when it comes to listening to and understanding what you have to say.

The people you meet in a support group will be able to provide you with advice and understanding that you can only get from someone in the know.

View it as part of your weekly routine and ensure that if you have to organise for someone to be there with your partner that they understand how important it is for you. It's harder to change your mind about your "me time" at the last moment if you have a set event to go to each week.

When the Disease Progresses

Go and look at nursing homes and look at the extras they offer and the added company they can provide. Your partner's condition will get worse, and there's no set timescale for when that will happen. The worsening of the condition will be a gradual process and will not happen overnight. It is likely that you have slowly begun to make changes both in the house and in your lifestyle.

Discuss with your loved one what they want to happen and how they want to be cared for in the later stages. If you feel that it would be easier, and would cause fewer problems particularly with other family members, write down these wishes and keep them safe. It's best to be prepared, though you shouldn't focus entirely on what is to come.

Most of all, get rid of any guilt you have. Just do what you can and be there for them. There's no way of knowing if you have years left, or just a few months. Try and take a step back when making decisions.

Tell your children what your partner's wishes are – if you have children – and sit down as a family to discuss them while there's still plenty of time.

It's best to make any difficult decisions while your partner is well enough to make them with you, so try to talk about things in advance. Tell your children what your partner's wishes are – if you have children – and sit down as a family to discuss them while there's still plenty of time. Take the time to put plans into motion when signs begin to show that the disease is moving into its next stage.

As tempting as it may be, don't ignore the symptoms. Respect your partner's wishes when the time comes to put them into action. There may well come a time when you need help, as much as you want to keep caring for your partner at home. If you aren't sure about the best thing to do, try to get advice from a range of different people to get as many different insights as possible.

In the relatives of people in the later stages of dementia, one of the most common and destructive emotions you're likely to find is guilt. This will do neither you nor your partner any good. It's a negative, unproductive emotion, so try your best to avoid falling into its trap at all costs.

Summing Up

- Many couples find it difficult to deal with changes to one partner's personality, so it's very common for a marriage to deteriorate long before Alzheimer's is even diagnosed. In these cases, it can be a real relief to find out what's actually wrong.

- Following your partner's diagnosis, try to get together as much information about the condition as you can. There's so much information out there about why sufferers do things a certain way and why different changes take place. This can really reduce frustration by helping you understand that there's reasoning behind even the smallest changes.

- Understand how important it is that you get some time to yourself regularly. Continue with any interests and pastimes you enjoy, and try to find a carer's support group where you can talk about your experiences.

- The time will come when the condition worsens. While you should focus on the present day, you should not ignore the inevitable. Be prepared and talk about it together. Know what your partner wants.

- Be aware of the signs that the disease is worsening and be prepared for them.

- It can seem as if you have lost the person you love. You should not focus on the aspects of the person you have lost but on what you have now. There can still be fun and laughter.

10

When a Parent is Diagnosed

It can send shockwaves through the entire family if one of your parents is diagnosed with Alzheimer's disease. There may be a period of denial, with some relatives not agreeing with the diagnosis and pushing for a second opinion. The diagnosis can be especially shocking to those who don't live with the individual and haven't been there to see the warning signs for themselves.

Trying to maintain your own life can be hard as the responsibilities increase. Often one person takes on most of the care. This can cause no end of resentment and bad feeling in families, often leading to relationship breakdowns.

It may begin to feel as though you've swapped roles and become your parent's parent if you're the person who ends up caring for them. This can be strange and uncomfortable for both of you – your parent may resent you for treating them like a child, while you might resent the reversal of roles or feel shocked that you've found your new position comes so naturally/unnaturally to you.

If one sibling takes complete control right from the start, others can begin to accept this as the norm. If you are an only child, it can seem unfair that you are left to deal with everything and you may wish that you had a sibling to share the responsibility. Suddenly having to worry about someone else all the time can be stressful if you're used to being a very independent person.

In the later stages of the disease, it's common for friction to occur within families. As more care is needed and it becomes harder for one person to cope, that person may begin to look to their family for more assistance. A more sensible course of action is to try and share the load right from the start.

However, the idealistic situation of every family member working together and taking it in turns to care for your parent won't always happen, even in larger and seemingly close families. Some family members will be happy to let you do everything while they stay out of the situation, while others might genuinely live too far away to help out much, or have a busy job or young children who take up all of their time.

It can be a good idea to try and resolve any tensions before they really kick in. People's lives grow and change so if someone really doesn't seem to have time to help at first, give them time to make room before suggesting again that they chip in. Ensure that they understand the work and responsibility involved and that it should really be shared.

Don't create a dispute between yourself and the rest of the family, but try to make it clear that you would appreciate their assistance. Try your best to get your brothers and sisters to involve themselves in supporting your parents and helping with tricky decisions.

Helping Mum and Dad

Children can be a really positive escape from the mundane and can be particularly good for those with depression. Frequency and length of visits will be dependent on many factors, including the age and activity level of the child as well as what the person with Alzheimer's can cope with. For visits to go well, the child must enjoy visiting and not get bored. This is easy enough to judge and should not be ignored.

The grandparent may well forget the child's name but children are amazingly adaptable and may well find it funny. When it comes to spending time with young children, people with Alzheimer's disease are no different to any other elderly person. A visit from a child can really bring a lot of pleasure. Seeing someone's face light up when your child walks into the room can be a real boost for the whole family.

When it comes to reality orientation, grandchildren can be especially helpful. Their visits can act as a trigger for the individual to help them understand how they fit into the family and who their loved ones are.

By discussing the child and related details, you can indirectly get your parent to think about this without making it seem like you're there to therapise them. Bringing your child on visits may not always be appropriate, but if you judge every situation as it arises you should get a clear idea of when a visit from a grandchild will and won't be a positive experience (for all parties).

Keep in mind that visits from loud or rowdy children may simply upset or irritate the individual, as the noise and activity level can get too much.

Make sure you're also taking into account the needs of the child in question. For example, if the person with Alzheimer's has issues with incontinence, this may confuse or distress the child, so it may be best to keep visits on the shorter side to avoid this situation.

Making a memory book, or life story book, is another positive activity that you can do with the whole family. This is a personal account of all the people and things that are important to the individual. You can buy ready made life story books designed for you to insert pictures or you can use a scrap book and make your own. Each picture acts as a reason to talk about that person or place and topics leading off from that.

The memory book can be a fun prompt for the person with Alzheimer's, allowing them to go through the book with someone and tell them all about the people and places in each photo. This can encourage their brain to remember the past and the people who are important to them. As the family begins to lose their link to the past, the memory book can also be a nice keepsake for younger family members.

Ways You Can Help – Questions

Families are often at a loss over whether to go along with what the person thinks or to correct them. When someone in your family has Alzheimer's, how do you know what are the right and wrong things to do?

This section discusses some of the most common questions a relative might have.

Making a memory book, or life story book, is another positive activity that you can do with the whole family. This is a personal account of all the people and things that are important to the individual.

My mother refers to my dad as if he is still alive. Should I tell her the truth or go along with pretending?

Protecting a person with Alzheimer's will sometimes involve telling the odd white lie. If your mum is going to react as if she is hearing the news for the first time and is going to upset and grieve for your dad, then it is not a good idea to put her through that. Try thinking about whether the news that her husband is dead will upset her or not.

If possible, try to avoid telling lies or the truth in this situation by sidestepping the issue.

If my father gets me and my sister confused, should I correct him?

In situations like this, try to think about trigger points. Will knowing the difference be of benefit to your father? Will telling him help him to remember other facts about your family. If the answer is yes and telling him isn't likely to upset him, then correcting him may be your best bet.

If you think it will upset him, however, don't bother bringing it up. Upsetting your father won't make things better, and won't stop him from forgetting again in the future.

My uncle is now at the point where he can't manage on his own but none of the family can take him in. He refuses to go into a home. What can we do?

Keep trying to talk him round and try to convince him that it is in his best interests. You can't force your uncle to go into a home, but you can try and help him realise that a nursing home is probably the best place for him. Getting a social worker or CPN to talk to him may also be a good idea if you feel you aren't getting anywhere.

I'm worried my father is going to hurt himself as he's had a few falls already. What can I do, other than trying to remove obstacles in the house?

If you contact an occupational therapist, they'll be able to conduct an assessment in your home and advise you on what to do. There are a few things they may ask you to consider. For example, try to make sure that every room in your house is properly lit with no dark corners by making sure all of the light bulbs are working and producing enough light.

One of the most common causes of falls is badly fitting footwear. Your father's risk of tripping up will be increased if he's wearing shoes that are the wrong size. Unsuitable footwear is also an issue, for example shoes with laces can cause falls if the person forgets to tie them.

There has been much research conducted into how the mind works when someone develops dementia. Take a look at the carpets on the floor of each room. One thing that researchers have found is that people with Alzheimer's can become disoriented by looking at patterned and swirly carpets.

Key Points to Consider

Someone with Alzheimer's disease may become upset and worried about their situation as their condition progresses. They may want to talk about these concerns in the earlier stages of the disease. Caring for someone with Alzheimer's is more than just about caring for their physical needs. It is important that you take the time to sit down and listen rather than dismissing their concerns.

Avoid speaking to the person as if they are a child and, whenever possible, speak with them, not about them. Always make them feel valued and give them the respect they are due. Support your parent in expressing their feelings, and show them that you are there for them.

As the disease progresses, it is all too easy to start thinking of the person differently. Keep in mind that these people are individuals, and are more than just their condition. This is not simply someone who suffers from Alzheimer's – this is your mum, dad, uncle or friend, who has memories and interests and ideas, and who is a person in their own right.

Respect the person's privacy and dignity. For example, if they develop issues with incontinence, find a way to deal with it in a sensitive and respectful manner.

No matter how far the disease progresses, don't allow yourself to act like they're not in the room. Don't talk to someone else about them while they're sitting there. They are a person and they can hear you.

Try to understand why your parent has started to act a certain way, or do certain things. Become an expert in your parent's condition and needs.

Case Study

"My dad never got on with his sister's husband, but was always civil with him until the last few years when my aunt was diagnosed with Alzheimer's. My dad refused to recognise that she had developed this condition, and wouldn't accept the diagnosis. Eventually, it got to the point where my aunt could no longer visit or even write letters. My dad came to the conclusion that this was all a conspiracy cooked up by his brother-in-law to keep him away from his sister.

"All this rage ended up affecting my own relationship with my father. I tried to talk to him about Alzheimer's, but he would always just get really angry with me.

"My aunt died a few years back, and my father still hasn't accepted her condition." – Deborah, age 56.

Summing Up

- A diagnosis of Alzheimer's disease can come as a major shock, and can cause real damage to family relationships.

- When you're caring for a parent with Alzheimer's, it can feel like the roles are reversing and you're becoming your parent's parent.

- People with Alzheimer's can find visits from grandchildren very therapeutic. The situation and the age of the child will determine how much you tell them and how you carry out these visits.

- Avoid speaking to the person with Alzheimer's as if they are a child, and make sure you are giving them the respect they deserve.

- Consider making a life story book – both to aid the person's memory and as a lasting reminder for the whole family.

- Often, one person ends up doing most of the caring. This can lead to resentment between siblings.

- From the start, try to ensure that one person is not left to do everything.

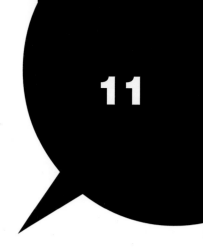

11

The Future

Y ou can't help worrying about the future, even if you know it's best to live in the present. You may find it puts your mind at rest if you plan what you want in the future. As the disease progresses, try to leave yourself free of worry by dealing with your affairs well in advance.

Is There Anything to Look Forward To?

People who have been diagnosed with Alzheimer's often worry about what will happen when they become too ill to look after themselves. Reassessing life and what the future holds isn't always that appealing, so it can easily feel like Alzheimer's is forcing your hand a little. Alzheimer's has no life plan and nobody can tell you when things will progress or how long you have before you reach the final stages.

Everyone wants to know how long they have, and in the majority of cases there's simply no way of knowing. It's best to focus on the present to a certain extent, as it's not possible to plan for the future in any real detail. However, there are some plans which require no time scales and you can always put these into place. The Alzheimer's Society encourages people to put together an advanced statement.

An advance statement can be used to lay out any aspect of your future social or health care, such as where you'd like to be cared for (at home, in a nursing home, hospital or hospice), whether you prefer baths or showers, who will look after any pets you have and how you want your spiritual and religious beliefs reflected in your care.

A living will, or advance decision, allows you to decide in advance what care you want to receive (if any) in the event that you are no longer able to care for yourself, and gives you the right to refuse any life-sustaining treatments if you do not wish to receive them. (Note: This is not the same thing as assisted suicide, which is illegal in the UK.)

Be sure to discuss your advance statement and advance decision with your GP to make sure that they are valid and don't contain any conflicting statements. Be sure that your family also know what it contains so that they know what to expect.

It's best to review both of your statements regularly in case you want to make any changes, and to leave an up-to-date copy with your lawyer and a close relative. For information on what the statements should contain, contact the Alzheimer's Society.

As we've already discussed, many people find it a real relief to know they've dealt with their financial affairs.

You can find out what services are available in your area, and what plans you can put in place for when you're too ill to care for yourself, by talking to a CPN or social worker.

A living will, or advance decision, allows you to decide in advance what care you want to receive (if any) in the event that you are no longer able to care for yourself, and gives you the right to refuse any life-sustaining treatments if you do not wish to receive them.

What Is Being Done to Look for a Cure?

The words 'Alzheimer's cure' hits the headlines regularly and millions of people read on hoping that it will say that cure has definitely been found and that the destruction it causes can now be reversed. We're yet to receive this piece of news, but that doesn't stop us from hoping we someday will.

Since Alois Alzheimer discovered the disease over 100 years ago, we've certainly come a long way. That said, it sometimes seems as though we've made no progress at all. This does not mean that little is being done to achieve this aim. Much work is still needed, but great leaps have been made over the last 30-40 years.

Compared with £289 for each cancer patient, £11 per head is currently spent each year in the UK to research a cure for Alzheimer's, according to the Alzheimer's Research Trust. It doesn't seem to matter that similar numbers of people are affected by the two diseases.

The late Terry Pratchett, a bestselling author of fantasy novels, met with prime minister Gordon Brown in November 2008, presenting him with a petition containing 18,000 signatures to demand more funding for Alzheimer's research. The disease was kept firmly in the headlines for some time as a result of Pratchett's diagnosis, and the author did everything he could to lobby for a cure up until his death in 2015.

More recently, dementia and mental illness have both been thrown into the spotlight by the death of Robin Williams, who took his own life in 2014 following a long struggle with depression and a diagnosis of dementia with Lewy bodies.

There have been many trials with positive results, too many to name here, but still nothing concrete. An optimistic way of looking at things is that with each research trial, more is discovered about the disease and how it works. Research released in 2018 prompted a series of headlines suggesting we could expect a cure for Alzheimer's "within the next six years", but similar five-year promises were being made over a decade ago.

The work to find a successful cure is ongoing, despite the low level of funding. Every piece of research is like a jigsaw piece, according to the Alzheimer's Research Trust, and each piece will contribute to the completion of the final puzzle.

Ongoing Research

To help understand the disease we need to know as much as possible about its causes, why certain changes happen and what exactly happens to the brain. If we want to find a cause and a cure for Alzheimer's, research is mandatory.

With an ageing population, Alzheimer's is going to affect more people, so there will be an even greater need for a cure. Alzheimer's Research UK links 15 research centres throughout the UK. Since 1992, Alzheimer's Research UK (formerly Alzheimer's Research Trust) has invested over £101,233,175 into research projects that look into new ways for dementia to be cured, treated or prevented.

One funded project helped scientists to identify routes to potential treatments when it found a DNA link to Parkinson's disease and Lewy body disease. Another offered hope for a potential blood test to diagnose the disease when it identified markers in the blood for the development of Alzheimer's. Another project was able to identify 40 compounds which showed potential for the development of Alzheimer's drugs by screening 1.5 million different compounds.

In their 2018 annual review, Alzheimer's Research UK announced that the UK Dementia Research Institute was now running six separate centres, with teams of researchers working across the UK. Scientists at the UK DRI were making progress on more than two dozen different projects, with discoveries being made in using brain scans to identify early changes in the brain before Alzheimer's symptoms have developed.

Alzheimer's Research UK are currently funding a number of studies on Alzheimer's, including one that assesses the biological consequences of a potential Alzheimer's treatment, one which aims to identify targets to tackle brain inflammation, and a study on hallucinations in dementia with Lewy bodies.

Research is ongoing, with a number of other research institutes and universities across the country conducting their own studies on the disease. Without a doubt, we are slowly building up a clearer picture of the disease by learning more about its progression and causes, but there's no way of knowing how close to finding a cure we really are.

Case Studies

Eric, aged 53

"Caring for someone with Alzheimer's has affected my freedom to a certain extent. Two years ago, my mother was diagnosed with Alzheimer's at the age of 81. At the moment it is still early days but she is happy enough and is fortunate enough to have plenty of company. She still has her own house but I don't let her sleep there. She can still feed and wash herself, and she isn't incontinent, so she's very capable in many respects.

"She spends time in her own house during the day, but eats and sleeps at my place. I think she enjoys the freedom, and it's only 5 minutes down the road. It means I can still go out and do my shopping and things, even if I can't just go away and leave her on her own.

"We're learning the importance of living life in the moment."

Marian, aged 66

"My father became very forgetful when he developed dementia, and became increasingly dependent on me. I was working full-time and found it very difficult to cope. I felt I was chasing my tail most of the time. I wanted to have him at my house but he wanted to take the bus home – something he had never done from my house. At one point, he accused me of stealing from him and I was really upset about that for a while.

"The more I did for my father, the more my own family had to take second place. Until my sister, Fiona, contacted the Adams Agency, I was able to get very little support. They sent someone in to make him a light lunch and help him. The service was very helpful, but we did have to pay for it. Sometimes he refused to let them in, though, so that could be difficult.

"My father started naming parts of the city he'd lived in before he married my mother if anyone asked him where he lived.

"Eventually, I took my father to be assessed. The specialists told me I should find somewhere that he could go for respite, and ideally somewhere he could stay permanently. It took us a while, but we were eventually able to find a residential home that suited his needs."

Greg, aged 67

"My wife's entire personality has changed since her diagnosis. We have been through a lot in our lives, like business problems and divorce, but nothing can compare to the despair and anger I feel with this disease. Dementia changes the whole character of the person. It's nothing like the other awful diseases out there, like cancer. She's turned into a miserable, touchy, withdrawn person who's frightened of everything, but she used to be so happy, talkative and positive!

"I would say she was born to talk – sometimes too much. She was once renowned for her communication skills, and always loved a chat.

"We have been told that her disease is not following the normal pattern – it has severely affected her language skills but she can still find her way around on the train by herself. We can't understand each other anymore – we're like two strangers living together.

"One of our daughters has taken to totally ignoring us (she doesn't even phone!), but the other has been very supportive."

Staying Positive

How do you stay positive when you have been diagnosed with a disease which, as yet, has no cure? When you have a condition like Alzheimer's disease, it can be pretty difficult to stay positive. It's the best way of coping with the disease, though, so it's important that you find a way. It can be very difficult to pull yourself out of the depression that you risk falling into if you lose your positive attitude.

As we've said, it's much more difficult to make yourself stay positive than it is to tell someone else to. But there are some tips that can help. Many of us go through life with plans for what we will do in the future but never get round to it. Don't blame yourself and don't blame the advice you were given or not given – just forget blaming altogether.

Be ready for the changes which may occur but don't focus on them. Enjoy life and appreciate what you have got. Reading the many newspaper reports on suggested causes and what we could have done in the past will not help and is not a proactive way of living your life. Letting go of any blame you hold should be your first step. It's not possible to rule out your potential to develop Alzheimer's by living a healthy life, eating your greens or keeping your mind active.

It's very unlikely that you could have avoided this condition, so there's no point in blaming yourself for it.

Make changes that will allow you to continue enjoying life and aim to get as much out of every day as you can. Keep your sense of humour or develop a stronger one. If you can't find the dishes because they are in the washing machine – laugh. Next time you ask someone what day it is only to discover you have already asked this at least 10 times, laugh.

If you did something as silly as this and you didn't have Alzheimer's you would laugh, so why not now? The second tip is to remember the importance of laughing. Just keep laughing. There are plenty of things you can find funny in your day-to-day life. You don't need to take things seriously all the time! There's absolutely nothing wrong with laughing at the things your condition makes you do.

Make sure you are enjoying life, and take each day as it comes. Do everything you want to do, provided health and circumstance allow it.

Alzheimer's is too hard to predict and does not follow a certain path. Try not to become a fortune-teller. You shouldn't try to predict the future – and you won't be able to if you do try. Just stick with enjoying today.

The most important tip is to remember that while Alzheimer's is part of your life now, it doesn't define who you are and doesn't change what you have achieved.

Summing Up

- Don't focus on the future, but make sure you're ready for it. Making up an advanced statement is a good way of taking the pressure off later on.

- The research that's happening today is constantly moving us slowly towards a cure. While we haven't found one yet, we'll get there eventually.

- Staying positive is vital. Try to enjoy every day, and keep your sense of humour. Keep in mind that your condition is only a tiny part of who you are. Make the most of every little thing, and live for today.

- Much research is being conducted into causes and prevention, helping us to understand the whole make-up of the disease.

- Alzheimer's research is severely underfunded but much work is still being done.

Sources

Advance decision (living will) - NHS
www.nhs.uk/conditions/end-of-life-care/advance-decision-to-refuse-treatment

Advance statement about your wishes - NHS
www.nhs.uk/conditions/end-of-life-care/advance-statement

Alzheimer's Research UK Annual Review 2018
http://review. Alzheimer'sresearchuk.org

Could vitamin E slow dementia? - NHS
www.nhs.uk/news/neurology/could-vitamin-e-slow-dementia

Do "Brain-Training" Programs Work?
https://journals.sagepub.com/stoken/rbtfl/hK6Y5zBl1Rv.M/full

Facts for the media
www. Alzheimer's.org.uk/about-us/news-and-media/facts-media

Ginkgo biloba and stroke risk - NHS
www.nhs.uk/news/food-and-diet/ginkgo-biloba-and-stroke-risk

How much research we fund - Dementia Statistics Hub
www.dementiastatistics.org/statistics/how-much-research-we-fund

Managing your affairs and enduring power of attorney - nidirect
www.nidirect.gov.uk/articles/managing-your-affairs-and-enduring-power-attorney

Memory clinics - Dementia Statistics Hub
www.dementiastatistics.org/statistics/memory-clinics

Online dementia training for GPs and practice nurses
www. Alzheimer's.org.uk/online-dementia-training-gps-and-practice-nurses

Research projects - Alzheimer's Research UK
www. Alzheimer'sresearchuk.org/our-research/research-projects

Speaking of Psychology: Protecting your aging brain
www.apa.org/research/action/speaking-of-psychology/aging-brain

Help List

ACAS

www.acas.org.uk

Acas (Advisory, Conciliation and Arbitration Service) provides free and impartial information and advice to employers and employees on all aspects of workplace relations and employment law. "We support good relationships between employers and employees which underpin business success. But when things go wrong we help by providing conciliation to resolve workplace problems."

Age UK

www.ageuk.org.uk

Email: contact@ageuk.org.uk

England

Address: Tavis House, 1-6 Tavistock Square, London WC1H 9NA

Tel: 0800 169 80 80

Wales

Address: Ground Floor, Mariners House, Trident Court, East Moors Road, Cardiff CF24 5TD

Tel: 029 2043 1555

Scotland

Address: Causewayside House, 160 Causewayside, Edinburgh, EH9 1PR

Tel: 0845 125 9732

Northern Ireland

Address: 3 Lower Crescent, Belfast, BT7 1NR

Tel: 028 9024 5729

Formerly Age Concern and Help the Aged, Age UK is the country's largest charity dedicated to helping everyone make the most of later life. They provide advice, help and companionship to the older people who need it the most.

Alzheimer's Disease International

www.alz.co.uk

Address: 64 Great Suffolk Street, London, SE1 0BL

Tel: 020 79810880

Email: info@alz.co.uk

Alzheimer's Disease International is the international federation of Alzheimer's organisations all over the world. They provide advice and support as well as details of research and statistics.

Alzheimer's Research UK

www. Alzheimer'sresearchuk.org

Address: 3 Riverside, Granta Park, Cambridge CB21 6AD

Tel: 0300 111 5555

Email: enquiries@ Alzheimer'sresearchuk.org

Formerly Alzheimer's Research Trust, this organisation's scientists have been behind some of the biggest breakthroughs in dementia research. They're working to bring us closer to a future free of the damage, heartbreak and fear associated with dementia.

Alzheimer Scotland

www.alzscot.org

Address: 160 Dundee Street, Edinburgh EH11 1DQ

Tel: 0131 243 1453

Email: info@alzscot.org

Alzheimer Scotland is Scotland's leading dementia organisation. They provide a wide range of personalised and innovative support services and campaign for the rights of people with dementia and their families.

Alzheimer's Society

www. Alzheimer's.org.uk

Address: 43-44 Crutched Friars, London EC3N 2AE

Tel: 0330 333 0804

Email: (Contact through website – www. Alzheimer's.org.uk/form/email-a-question-to-the-helpline)

Alzheimer's Society describes itself as "the only UK charity that campaigns for change, funds research to find a cure and supports people living with dementia today."

American Psychological Association

www.apa.org

Address: 750 First St. NE, Washington, DC 20002-4242

Tel: (800) 374-2721 | (202) 336-5500

Email: (Contact through website – www.apa.org/support/contact)

The American Psychological Association is "the leading scientific and professional organisation representing psychology in the United States, with more than 118,000 researchers, educators, clinicians, consultants and students as its members."

It no longer has an information page on memory training for Alzheimer's, but still has plenty of interesting articles that may come in handy.

Carer's Allowance Unit

www.gov.uk/carers-allowance

Address: Mail Handling Site A, Wolverhampton WV98 2AB

Tel: 0800 731 0297

Email: cau.customer-services@dwp.gsi.gov.uk

Find out if your carers could access the Carer's Allowance. More information is available on the Directgov website.

Carers Trust

www.carers.org

Address: 32-36 Loman Street, London SE1 0EH

Tel: 0300 772 9600

Email: info@carers.org

"Carers Trust is a major charity for, with and about carers."

They're working to improve the services, information and support available to those who provide unpaid care to friends and family members who are unable to care for themselves.

Dementia Research Centre

www.ucl.ac.uk/drc/

Address: Box 16, The National Hospital for Neurology and Neurosurgery, Queen Square, London, WC1N 3BG

Tel: +44 (0)20 3448 4773

Email: cognitivedisordersclinic@uclh.org

The Dementia Research Centre is one of the UK's leading centres for clinical research into dementia. It also trials new drugs to slow the progression of Alzheimer's.

Disability Service Centre

www.gov.uk/disability-benefits-helpline

Address: Warbreck House, Warbreck Hill, Blackpool, Lancashire, FY2 0YE

Tel: 0800 121 4600 (DLA helpline)

See the GOV.UK website for detail son the Disability Living Allowance and the Attendance Allowance or contact the helpline for more information.

GOV.UK

www.gov.uk

This is the best place to find information about government services in your area.